T0207128

Cicatricial Alopecia

Vera Price
Paradi Mirmirani (EDs.)

Cicatricial Alopecia

An Approach to Diagnosis and Management

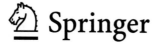

Springer

Editors
Vera Price
Professor, Department of Dermatology
University of California, San Francisco
San Francisco, California 94115
USA
pricev@derm.ucsf.edu

Paradi Mirmirani
Staff Physician
Department of Dermatology,
University of California, San Francisco
San Francisco, California 94115,
USA
and
Department of Dermatology
Case Western Reserve University
Cleveland, OH
USA
and
Department of Dermatology
The Permanente Medical Group,
975 Sereno Drive, Vallejo,
California 94589,
USA
paradi.mirmirani@kp.org

ISBN 978-1-4939-4112-4   ISBN 978-1-4419-8399-2 (eBook)
DOI 10.1007/978-1-4419-8399-2
Springer New York Dordrecht Heidelberg London

Springer is part of Springer Science+Business Media (www.springer.com)

Preface

There have been several recent reviews published of the primary cicatricial alopecias, so why was this monograph produced? We felt there was a need for a richly-illustrated and practical text that would be a teaching vehicle primarily for dermatology residents and interested dermatology colleagues. We realize that hair loss in general is not a topic on the curriculum of all dermatology departments, and cicatricial alopecia (scarring alopecia) in particular is frequently not covered.

At the University of California, San Francisco, we have held grand rounds dedicated entirely to the scarring alopecias. Introductory lectures are given highlighting clinical and histologic aspects, current treatments, and a summary of new research. In the patient viewing session, patients with characteristic features of each of the predominantly lymphocytic and neutrophilic cicatricial alopecias are presented. By "immersing" residents and colleagues in the topic of cicatricial alopecias, they have been able to envision a more global and systematic view of these disorders. The feedback has been tremendous: "I finally got it!"

In writing this monograph, we sought to replicate such a teaching session, and the information is presented as though the reader was "shadowing" us in the clinic. Each disease chapter is introduced with a clinical scenario of a patient, along with relevant clues for making the diagnosis. The discussion section follows and includes multiple photographs and take-away pearls to provide practical information needed to diagnose, manage, and counsel the patient. The suggested reading is not meant to be an exhaustive literature review, but rather a list of a few salient references. The voices of the patients can be heard in the chapter written by patients who tell of their frustrations in being undiagnosed by doctor after doctor, and untreated or mistreated for years. Our goal is to put the cicatricial alopecias on the center stage for dermatology residents and colleagues, because dermatologists may be the only physicians who can diagnose and treat these patients.

San Francisco, CA, USA   Vera Price
Vallejo, CA, USA   Paradi Mirmirani

Acknowledgments

We have been privileged to care for and follow many patients with cicatricial alopecia, and are grateful to all of them for giving us the first-hand opportunity to learn about these conditions. Our patients emphasize how much research is needed to increase our understanding and improve our current treatments, and we dedicate this monograph to them. We thank the six patients who shared their personal experiences with cicatricial alopecia in Chapter 10.

We are indebted to the Cicatricial Alopecia Research Foundation (CARF) for changing the landscape for these diseases. The Foundation was associated with the production of this monograph and is an indispensable resource for patients and doctors alike. We are grateful to the many CARF volunteers who provided valuable contributions during various phases of this monograph. We also thank Sheila Belkin, CARF's CEO, for coordinating the patient chapter and for her encouragement throughout.

We would like to thank Dr. Bruce Wintroub for his ongoing support of our interest in cicatricial alopecia. He has been instrumental in fostering collaborations that have moved our work and knowledge forward. We are grateful to many individuals whose help has been invaluable in creating the monograph. Dr. Tim McCalmont guided us through countless scalp biopsies and wrote the chapter on dermatopathology. He and Dr. Phil LeBoit both continue to enlighten us about the histopathology of cicatricial alopecia. Dr. Aman Samrao worked diligently throughout the entire production, and her assistance was indispensable in handling tables, figures, clinical images, and whatever was asked of her. Dr. Jeffrey Donovan gave valuable editorial input and assisted with assembling the references. Dr. Tim Berger helped to update many concepts and to remove old baggage from this field; we greatly appreciate his interest in clarifying the lexicon. We thank Canfield Scientific for generously giving us the use of their Nikon camera. We are indebted to Dr. Sarah Cipriano and Leslie Chau for their expert technical and administrative support. Finally, we gratefully acknowledge the major contribution of Dr. Pratima Karnik whose molecular studies have pioneered a breakthrough in understanding the crucial role of the sebaceous gland in normal hair growth and in the pathogenesis of cicatricial alopecia. We also wish to acknowledge Dr. Kurt Stenn, who for many prior years had advocated further study of the sebaceous gland and its role in hair growth and hair loss.

Contents

Contributors

Vera Price, MD, FRCP(C)
Professor, Department of Dermatology,
University of California, San Francisco, San Francisco,
California 94115, USA
pricev@derm.ucsf.edu

Paradi Mirmirani, MD
Staff Physician
Department of Dermatology,
University of California, San Francisco, San Francisco,
California 94115 USA; Department of Dermatology,
Case Western Reserve University, Cleveland, OH, USA;
Department of Dermatology, The Permanente Medical Group,
975 Sereno Drive, Vallejo, California 94589, USA
paradi.mirmirani@kp.org

Timothy H. McCalmont, MD
UCSF Dermatopathology Service, University of California,
San Francisco, 1701 Divisadero Street,
4th Floor, San Francisco, CA 94115, USA
tim.mccalmont@ucsf.edu

Sheila Belkin
CEO, Cicatricial Alopecia Research Foundation,
Los Angeles, CA 90064, USA
sheila@carfintl.org

Introduction

1

Vera Price and Paradi Mirmirani

How Are the Cicatricial Alopecias Classified?

Cicatricial alopecias (scarring alopecias) encompass a diverse group of inflammatory disorders that cause permanent destruction of the pilosebaceous unit and irreversible hair loss. They may be *primary or secondary*. In the primary group, the hair follicle is the target of a folliculocentric inflammatory attack that results in replacement of the follicle with fibrous tissue. The secondary scarring alopecias are the result of a non-folliculocentric process or external injury; follicular destruction is secondary and incidental, as in severe infections (kerion), infiltrations (tumors, metastatic cancer, sarcoid), physical injuries (thermal burns, radiation, traction). In this monograph, the focus is on the primary scarring alopecias.

A first step in improving dialogue among clinicians and investigators was the workshop on cicatricial alopecia sponsored by the North American Hair Research Society in 2001. This workshop proposed a working classification of the cicatricial alopecias based on the predominant cellular infiltrate, whether lymphocytic, neutrophilic, mixed, or absent in the end stage. After this workshop, the term *cicatricial* alopecia was adopted in the US, but the terms cicatricial and scarring are interchangeable. This classification continues to evolve, and a modified version is followed here (Table 1.1). The classification is currently used as a guide for selecting treatment.

Table 1.1 Working classification of primary cicatricial alopecia[a]

Lymphocytic group
  Lichen planopilaris
  Graham Little syndrome
  Frontal fibrosing alopecia
  Pseudopelade (Brocq)
  Central centrifugal cicatricial alopecia
  Chronic cutaneous lupus erythematosus[b]
  Keratosis follicularis spinulosa decalvans[b]

Neutrophilic group
  Folliculitis decalvans
  Tufted folliculitis

Mixed group
  Dissecting cellulitis[b]
  Folliculitis keloidalis[b]
End stage nonspecific group

[a]The above is a modification of the working classification of primary cicatricial alopecia which was proposed by the North American Hair Research Society in 2001. This modified classification is currently used by us as a guide for selecting treatment
[b]Not a primary cicatricial alopecia

What Are the Demographics of Patients with Cicatricial Alopecia?

The incidence of the cicatricial alopecias is not precisely known. The annual incidence rate of lichen planopilars (LPP) was reported in four tertiary hair research centers in the United States (Table 1.2). Annual incidence rate of LPP was defined as the percentage of new patients with biopsy-proven LPP and clinicopathologic correlation among all new patients with hair loss

V. Price and P. Mirmirani (eds.), *Cicatricial Alopecia: An Approach to Diagnosis and Management*,
DOI 10.1007/978-1-4419-8399-2_1, © Springer Science+Business Media, LLC 2011

seen over a 1-year period. In these four centers, the annual incidence of LPP varied from 1.15 to 7.59%, which attests to the relative rarity of LPP.

In a survey of 159 patients with cicatricial alopecia seen in the Dermatology Department, University of California, San Francisco between 2003 and 2005, the relative incidence of the various cicatricial alopecias, gender predisposition, racial incidence, and age of onset are shown in Figs. 1.1–1.4. However, the relative incidence of the various scarring alopecias shown in Fig. 1.1 represents patients who were referred to and seen in one geographic site (the

Table 1.2 Annual incidence of LPP in four tertiary hair research centers

Hair research center	All new hair loss cases (annual)	New LPP cases (annual)	LPP annual incidence rate (%)
University of California, San Francisco	580	44[a]	7.59
University of Pennsylvania	160	3	1.88
Baylor Hair Research and Treatment Center	433	5	1.15
Cleveland Clinic	55	3[b]	4.72

Reprinted from Ochoa BE, et al. Lichen planopilaris: annual incidence in four hair referral centers in the United States. J Am Acad Dermatol. 2008;58(2):353, copyright 2008, with permission from Elsevier
LPP Lichen planopilaris
[a]Includes cases of LPP, frontal fibrosing alopecia, and pseudopelade (Brocq)
[b]Number rounded up from 2.6

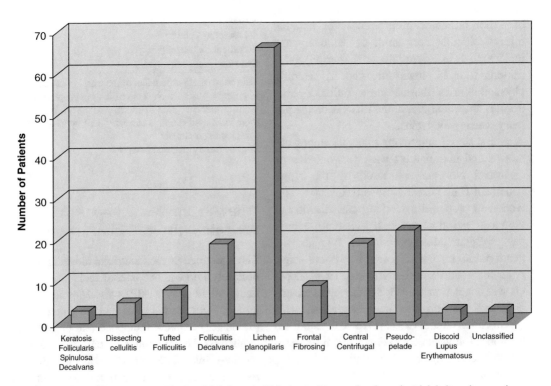

Fig. 1.1 Survey of 159 patients with cicatricial alopecia: Relative incidence of various cicatricial alopecias seen in one geographic site, the San Francisco Bay area, between 2003 and 2005. This incidence will vary at different geographic locations, depending on ethnic populations and referral patterns

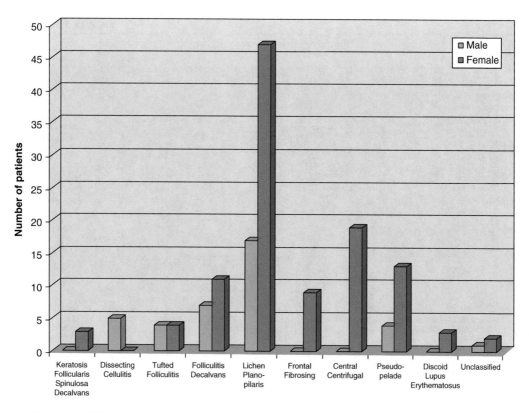

Fig. 1.2 Survey of 159 patients with cicatricial alopecia: gender predisposition

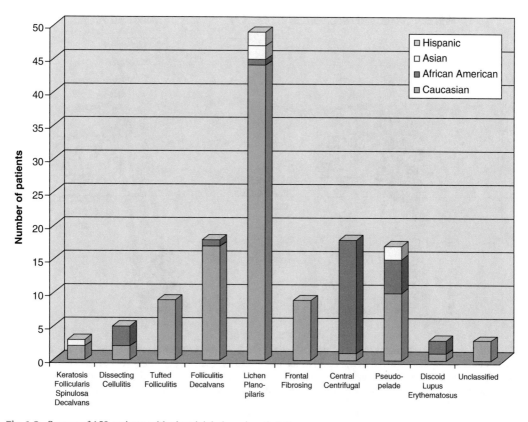

Fig. 1.3 Survey of 159 patients with cicatricial alopecia: ethnicity

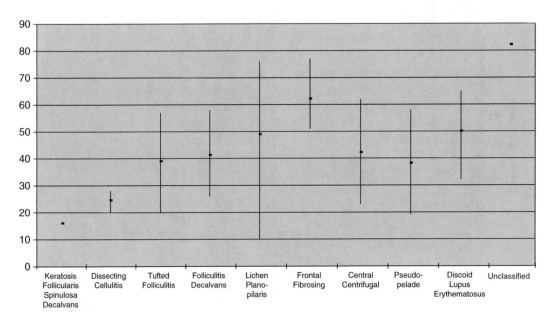

Fig. 1.4 Survey of 159 patients with cicatricial alopecia: age of onset

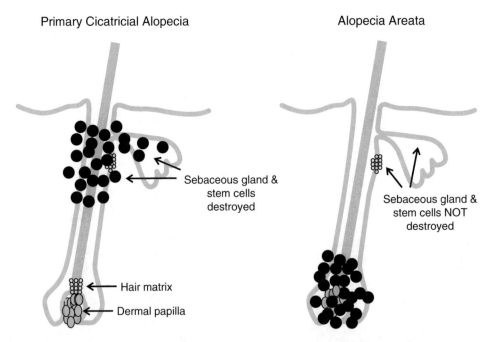

Fig. 1.5 In primary cicatricial alopecia, the inflammatory infiltrate is located around the upper part of the hair follicle around the infundibulum and isthmus and results in destruction of the hair follicle stem cells in the hair bulge and the sebaceous gland. Destruction of these structures leads to permanent hair loss. In contrast, alopecia areata is always potentially reversible because the inflammatory infiltrate is located around the hair bulb, and the sebaceous gland and the hair follicle stem cells are not affected. Courtesy of Jeff Donovan, MD

San Francisco Bay area). This incidence will vary widely at different geographic sites, depending on ethnic populations and referral patterns. The incidence of CCCA, for example, will increase with a higher population of African ancestry. At the same time, gender predisposition, racial incidence, and the age of onset are probably generally representative in Figs. 1.2–1.4.

Why Is Hair Loss in Cicatricial Alopecia Irreversible?

As with non-scarring alopecias such as androgenetic alopecia and alopecia areata, the cicatricial alopecias occur in healthy people and are not contagious. However, unlike androgenetic alopecia and alopecia areata, the hair loss is irreversible. Why is this?

The location of the perifollicular inflammatory infiltrate determines the irreversibility and reversibility of hair loss (Fig. 1.5). Destruction of the hair follicle stem cells and the sebaceous gland leads to permanent hair loss. For this reason, early and aggressive treatment of the scarring alopecias is key and is aimed at controlling the inflammatory infiltrate to minimize the extent of permanent hair loss.

Takeaway Pearls

> The terms cicatricial and scarring are interchangeable.
> Hair loss in cicatricial alopecia is irreversible because the inflammatory infiltrate is located around the infundibulum and isthmus and results in destruction of the hair follicle stem cells and the sebaceous gland.
> Alopecia areata is always potentially reversible because the inflammatory infiltrate is located around the hair bulb, and the hair follicle stem cells and sebaceous gland are not affected.

Suggested Reading

Ochoa BE, King LE Jr, Price VH. Lichen planopilaris: annual incidence in four hair research centers in the United States. J Am Acad Dermatol. 2004;50:25–32.

Olsen EA, Bergfeld WF, Cotsarelis G, et al. Summary of North American Hair Research Society (NAHRS)-sponsored Workshop on Cicatricial Alopecia, Duke University Medical Center, February 10 and 11, 2001. J Am Acad Dermatol. 2003;48:103–10.

Sperling LC, Cowper SE. The histopathology of primary cicatricial alopecia. Semin Cutan Med Surg. 2006;25:41–50.

Clinical Assessment of the Patient

2

Vera Price and Paradi Mirmirani

The patient with hair loss invariably complains "I am losing my hair," which can mean vastly different things in different patients. Every patient with hair loss should have the following baseline lab studies: CBC, TSH, ferritin, and vitamin D 25OH because you do not want to miss other possible contributing factors of hair loss.

Listen to the patient carefully. A common feedback from patients with cicatricial alopecia is that they have seen many doctors who listened only half heartedly and then sent them on their way. Taylor the consultation to uncover the chronology and specifics of each patient. It will vary depending on the problem and the patient.

The clinical examination begins as soon as you enter the room. Note the patient's hair style. Position all patients with hair problems in a chair, not on the exam table, in order to see the hair and scalp from above (unless you are a giraffe!). Good lighting is essential; ideally have a magnifying light and a dermatoscope. Before taking the full history, it often helps to look at the patient's scalp briefly to establish whether follicular ostia are present or absent. Diminished or absent ostia are the hallmark of cicatricial alopecia, and this helps to guide the history taking. If a cicatricial alopecia is suspected, a scalp biopsy is the essential first step in assessing the patient.

If Time Is Limited On the Initial Visit, Take the Scalp Biopsy On the First Visit, and Complete the Evaluation at Next Visit

Scalp Biopsy

Select an active hair-bearing area with positive anagen pull test (preferred but not essential); avoid old, bare, late-stage areas. Infiltrate biopsy site with 1% lidocaine with epinephrine, and *always* wait 10 min for maximum vasoconstriction. Position the patients sitting down, leaning over the examination table, and bracing their head with their hands (like The Thinker) (Fig. 2.1). If an assistant is available, have her hold gauze squares and Q-tip to help with hemostasis. Sample down to subcutis. Take one deep 4-mm punch biopsy in the direction of hair growth for horizontal sectioning and H & E staining, or two 4-mm punch biopsies for both horizontal and vertical sectioning (depending on the preference of your dermatopathologist). Close with 3-0 blue suture (helps in finding the site).

V. Price and P. Mirmirani (eds.), *Cicatricial Alopecia: An Approach to Diagnosis and Management*, DOI 10.1007/978-1-4419-8399-2_2, © Springer Science+Business Media, LLC 2011

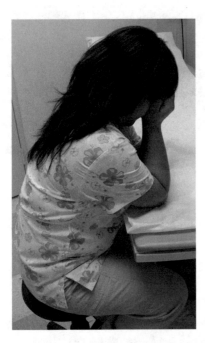

Fig. 2.1 Positioning for scalp biopsies and scalp injections. Have patients sit on a stool or a chair and lean over the exam table while bracing their chin or forehead with their hands ("The Thinker" position). If a biopsy is to be done on the occipital scalp, the patient may rest their head down on the table ("taking a nap on a school desk" position)

Evaluation of the Patient

History

- Establish the date of onset of the problem, rate of progression
- Assess symptoms: itching, pain, tenderness, burning
- Previous treatments?
- Has there been hair regrowth: this makes cicatricial alopecia unlikely
- Past health: document notable illnesses and infections prior to the onset
- Medications, including exogenous androgens, lipid-lowering drugs
- Diet – adequate protein? adequate calories?
- Hair care (chemicals, heat), hair cosmetics (more details in "Central Centrifugal Cicatricial Alopecia" in Chap. 6)

- Family history of similar problem: cicatricial alopecias rarely occur in family members except for CCCA. It is useful to establish whether androgenetic alopecia or alopecia areata exist in the family because more than one diagnosis may exist.

Examination

Have the patient remove hair pieces, pins, clips, braids, and note presence of hair extensions. A careful evaluation of the hair and scalp needs to be done (and is expected by the patient!). A thorough exam can be accomplished by serially parting the hair starting at the center part using the fingertips, or with a disposable comb, or with the wooden end of a Q-tip. The following assessment becomes automatic with practice:

Extent and Distribution of Hair Loss

- Is the scalp visible? Is the hair thinning apparent across the room?
- Diminished or absent ostia?
- Pattern and distribution: Focal patchy, patchy all over, or diffuse? central?
- Is the frontal hairline intact or is there frontal hairline recession with demarcation by photodamage below the original hairline?
- Is there hair thinning above the ears? Does it extend posteriorly to the occipital hairline?
- Distinguish traction hair loss from hairline recession due to frontal fibrosing alopecia and from alopecia areata. Take note if hairs outline the outer margins of the original hairline; this "fringe sign" is characteristic of traction alopecia (more details in Chap. 6: FFA and CCCA).
- Are there bare areas "bare as a baby's bottom"? (characteristic of alopecia areata)
- If the affected area is not completely bare, are the residual hairs terminal hairs, or fine textured and miniaturized (as in AA and AGA)?
- Eyebrows: Present or diminished?

Fig. 2.2 The Hair Card is a quick and easy way to distinguish new growth from broken or cut hair. In the figure shown, the distal ends are tapered (like the ends of eyelashes) indicating new growth. If the distal tips are blunt, this indicates the ends have been broken or cut. If some of the new short hair is thinner in diameter than the rest of the hair, it indicates miniaturization and may help to diagnose androgenetic alopecia

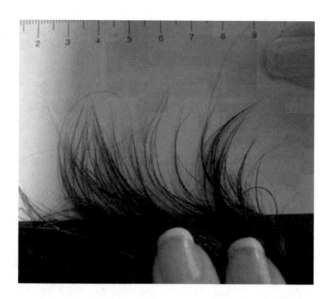

- Loss of hair at other sites: eyelashes, limbs, axillae, pubic area?
- Individual hairs in an affected area may be notably curly or kinky due to dermal fibrosis and subsequent follicular torsion.
- Photographs and measurements of the affected areas (if practical) are important for following the extent of hair loss. Photographs should include both close-up views and global views to identify nearby landmarks.
- The patient may have more than one condition. Assess the scalp for other conditions such as androgenetic alopecia and alopecia areata, which may coexist.

Scalp Assessment

- Follicular ostia are key: are they present, diminished, or absent? Are ostia patulous (distended) or dusky?
- Color of the affected scalp? Pink? Peach-colored? Skin-colored?
- "Fringe sign"?

---

[1]The Hair Card that we use refers to a 3 × 5 in. index card that is white on one side and black on the other side with a centimeter rule along one edge.

- Is there erythema? Is it perifollicular, in patches, all over?
- Scaling present? Is it perifollicular, in patches? all over?
- Are there pustules, crusts?
- Telangiectasia? atrophy?
- Hypo-, hyperpigmentation?

Hair Shaft Assessment

- The Hair Card[1]: Hair shafts and tips should be held against a contrasting white or black background, depending on the color of the hair, otherwise they may be difficult to see (Fig. 2.2 and Table 2.1).

Pull Test

- First, tell the patient that you are going to pull the hair.
- With the thumb and forefinger grasp a small swatch of hairs (about 30–40 hairs) close to the scalp. Gently but firmly slide the fingers away from the scalp at a 90° angle along the entire length of the hair swatch (Fig. 2.3). Do not tug or jerk.
- Negative pull test = 1–4 telogen hairs
- Positive pull test = 5 or more hairs

Table 2.1 The Hair Card

To assist in the examination and visualization of hair on the scalp, brows, and eyelashes, or elsewhere

What the Hair Card does:
Demonstrates miniaturized hair
Demonstrates new hair growth
Demonstrates broken hair and differentiates it from new growth

The ruler portion is used for:
Measuring length of new growth
Measuring temporal recession
Measuring dimensions of area of hair loss

How to use the Hair Card:
A good light source directed at the hair is essential when using the Hair Card
The black or white side is used to contrast with the color of the hair:
If dark hair is examined, use the white side
If blonde or white hair is examined, use the black side
To visualize the hair, place the blank (without any writing) portion of the card under or behind the hair to be examined.
    (The larger the blank portion of the card, the more useful it is)
Always place the Hair Card on the skin or as close to the skin surface as possible.

To demonstrate miniaturized hairs in androgenetic alopecia:
Select a thinning site on the scalp
Part the hair with your fingers
Place the Hair Card on the part you have created, directly on the scalp surface
A good light must be directed at the selected site
New short growth will be apparent against the contrasting color of the Hair Card, and miniaturized (thin) hair is easily
    identified and contrasted with new short growth of normal width (girth)

To differentiate new hair growth from broken (or cut) hair:
Place the Hair Card under the distal ends of the hair in question
New growth is easily identified because the distal ends are tapered or pointed
Broken hairs are easily identified because the distal ends are blunt or straight

To measure temporal recession:
Using the ruler side of the Hair Card, measure the distance from the lateral end of the brow to the apex of the
    temporal recession. In a male without temporal recession, the distance is approximately 6–6.5 cm

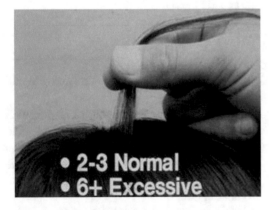

Fig. 2.3 How to do a pull test

- Where to pull?
- At the margin of a patch to see if the patch is active and about to progress
- In an unaffected scalp area to see if there is pending activity
- Pull on new growth to see if the new growth is "serious"
- Are the hair bulbs in a pull test anagen bulbs (A) or telogen bulbs (T)? The only time normal anagen hairs are easily extracted in a pull test is in active scarring alopecia. Normally, anagen hairs are not pulled out easily with a slow, firm pull. In primary cicatricial alopecia, the anagen/total ratio (A/T) is a useful indicator of active disease and of response to therapy.

Three situations in which anagen hairs may be easily extracted or affected:

1. Active primary cicatricial alopecia (Fig. 2.4)
2. Loose anagen syndrome (Fig. 2.5)
3. Anagen arrest during chemotherapy (Fig. 2.6)

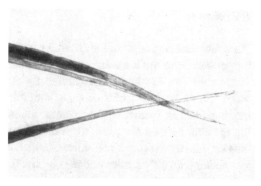

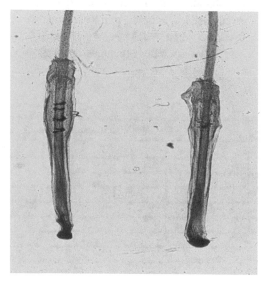

Fig. 2.6 Anagen arrest during chemotherapy. This is often inappropriately called anagen effluvium. Anagen hairs are not shed but are broken because during chemotherapy, mitotic activity in the matrix region of anagen hairs may be decreased resulting in transient narrowing of the hair shaft. When this narrow segment reaches the scalp surface, the hair breaks off

Fig. 2.4 The only time normal anagen hairs may be easily extracted in a pull test is in active cicatricial alopecia. This is a useful clinical indicator of active disease

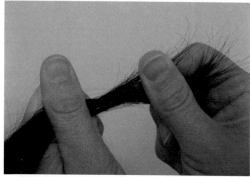

Fig. 2.7 How to do a tug test to demonstrate hair fragility

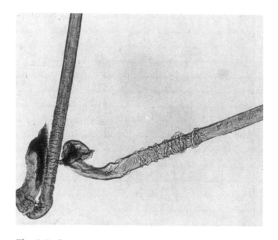

Fig. 2.5 Loose anagen hair is easily and painlessly pulled out in the loose anagen syndrome because the anchoring function of the inner root sheath is disturbed by structural abnormalities. Examination of the proximal shaft and hair bulb with light microscopy shows a distorted anagen bulb, a short twisted segment of the hair shaft immediately distal to the bulb, then a segment of shaft with the characteristic "ruffled" cuticle, and absent sheath

Tug Test

- Is the hair strong or fragile? Does it pull apart into little bits with a "tug test"? The "tug test" is the best way to demonstrate hair fragility.
- To perform the tug test, grasp a swatch of hairs with the fingers of one hand while the distal ends are plucked (as in plucking feathers) (Fig. 2.7). If the hair shaft is fragile or damaged, the hair will break into small bits. Any hair breakage constitutes an abnormality and should be noted.

Hair Mount

Put a few short segments of hair shaft, or broken bits of hair from the tug test, on a clean microscope slide; try to align them parallel to each other. Carefully drop 1 or 2 drops of mounting medium such as Permount ® or similar mounting medium on the hair; place a cover slip over the hairs and try to avoid air bubbles; exam under low power with a light microscope (Fig. 6.27).

Standardized Patient Flow Chart (Table 2.2)

At every visit, a flow chart is used to evaluate symptoms (pruritus, pain, burning), clinical signs (perifollicular scale, perifollicular erythema, erythema, pustules, crusting, pull test (anagen/total), and extent of hair loss. The chart is used to follow these three specific outcomes at each visit:

Table 2.2 Standardized flow chart

Name _____   Diagnosis _____

Date of visit				
A Pruritus				
B Pain				
C Burning				
D Erythema				
E Perifollicular erythema				
F Perifollicular scale				
*Crusting				
* Pustules				
Pull test: Anagen hairs/Total hairs				
Spreading				
Dimensions/Extent				
* Loss of follicular markings				
* Tufting				
* Telangiectasia				
* Atrophy				
* Pigment change				
* Other skin, nail, mucous membrane				
Labs CBC				
AST/ALT/Alk Phos				
G6PD				
Eye exam				
BUN/CR				
Blood Pressure				
Culture & Sensitivities				
Treatment/Comments				
Biopsy				
Photographs				
F/U visit				

Standardized flow chart is used at every visit of a patient with cicatricial alopecia. The flow chart allows easy evaluation of the patient's course over time, (otherwise who can remember?) and also makes sure that nothing has been omitted. Reprinted from Journal of the American Academy of Dermatology, Vol 62, Issue 3, Chiang C, et al. Hydroxychloroquine and lichen planopilaris: Efficacy and introduction of Lichen Planopilaris Activity Index scoring system, pgs 387–392, copyright 2010, with permission from Elsevier

Scale A–F: negative = -, questionable or mild = +/-, moderate = +, severe = ++
Spreading: Enter No, Uncertain, or Yes
*For these items: enter + or -

severity of symptoms, clinical disease activity including anagen positive pull test, and progression of hair loss. The flow chart allows easy evaluation of the patient's course and response to treatment over time and also makes sure nothing has been omitted during patient visits.

Takeaway Pearls

> Position all patients with hair problems in a chair, not on the exam table (unless you are a giraffe!).

> Good lighting is essential; ideally have a magnifying light.

> Before taking the full history, first look at the patient's scalp briefly to establish whether follicular ostia are present or absent.

> Diminished or absent ostia are the clinical hallmark of cicatricial alopecia.

> A history of hair regrowth makes cicatricial alopecia unlikely.

> If a cicatricial alopecia is suspected, a scalp biopsy is the essential first step in assessing the patient.

> If time is limited on the initial visit, take the scalp biopsy on the first visit and complete the evaluation at the next visit.

> Use a Hair Card for easy visualization of new growth, broken or cut hair, miniaturized hair.

> The only time normal anagen hairs are easily extracted in a pull test is in active scarring alopecia.

> A standardized flow chart is used at every visit to follow three specific outcome measures: the patient's symptoms, disease activity, and progression of hair loss.

> The flow chart allows easy evaluation of the patient's course over time (otherwise who can remember?)

Suggested Reading

Amor KT, Rashid RM, Mirmirani P. Does D matter? The role of vitamin D in hair disorders and hair follicle cycling. Dermatol Online J. 2010 Feb 15; 16(2):3.

Bikle DD. Vitamin D: newly discovered actions require reconsideration of physiologic requirements. Trends Endocrinol Metab. 2010;21(6):375–84.

Chiang C, Sah D, Cho BK, et al. Hydroxychloroquine and lichen planopilaris: Efficacy and introduction of lichen planopilaris activity index scoring system. J Am Acad Dermatol. 2010;62:387–92.

Mirmirani P, Willey A, Price VH. Short course of oral cyclosporine in lichen planopilaris. J Am Acad Dermatol. 2003;49:667–71.

Mirmirani P, Price VH, Karnik P. Decreased expression of follicular transglutaminases: A possible cause for loose anchoring of anagen hair in active primary cicatricial alopecia. J Invest Dermatol. 2008; 128S1:285.

Dermatopathology

Timothy H. McCalmont

The histopathological analysis of alopecia has represented a vexing area for clinicians and pathologists for as long as microscopes have existed. From the clinical perspective, there has been frustration that the pathologist or dermatopathologist could not provide them with a specific microscopical diagnosis that correlated with their clinical impression. For example, if the clinical morphology suggested pseudopelade but if the symptoms might also stem from follicular lichen planus (lichen planopilaris or LPP) (Fig. 3.1), why did the pathology report return with the simple generic diagnosis "scarring alopecia?"

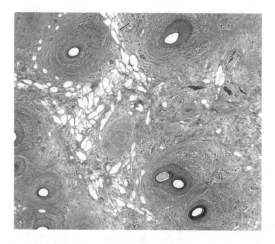

Fig. 3.1 Lymphocyte-mediated primary cicatricial alopecia (lichen planopilaris) at low magnification. There is a reduction in overall follicular density and a modest infiltrate can be seen around several folliculosebaceous units. A scarred follicular tract is prominent centrally in the frame. Perifollicular fibrosis is limited to the adventitial dermis and does not significantly involve the reticular dermis

From the histopathological perspective, there has been frustration that clinicians were overly attached to historically defined entities and reluctant to accept accurate yet less than specific interpretations that bridged standard diagnostic categories. For example, if the pathologist saw consecutive biopsies from two different patients with essentially identical histopathological attributes, yet one presented with clinical morphology favoring LPP while the other presented with morphology favoring frontal fibrosing alopecia (FFA), why would the clinician expect a different diagnosis for each specimen?

A breakthrough of sorts occurred at the University of California, San Francisco based upon histopathological analysis of biopsies of patients with cicatricial alopecia who presented in classical or stereotypical fashion (1). In this study, the microscopical attributes associated with cicatricial alopecia stratified into two dominant groups, which have come to be known as lymphocyte-mediated primary cicatricial alopecia (LMPCA) and neutrophil-mediated primary cicatricial alopecia (NMPCA). Stereotypical microscopical attributes that are associated with LMPCA and NMPCA are delineated in Table 3.1. Most classification schemes tend to be inherently flawed, and the division of cicatricial alopecia into lymphocyte-mediated and neutrophil-mediated categories is no exception, as it represents a practical yet imperfect solution to the problem. Imperfections include the fact that certain alopecic entities do not tidily pigeonhole as lymphocytic or neutrophilic in nature, and for biopsies from occasional patients with virtually any type of alopecia, especially biopsies obtained late in the course of disease, it can be challenging for the histopathologist or the investigator to make specific conclusions. In short, when evaluating a biopsy of late cicatricial disease, attempting to determine the precise events, whether lymphocyte-related or neutrophil-related, that elicited end-stage scarring can be difficult if not impossible.

LMPCA tends to be typified by a lymphocyte-rich infiltrate that elicits limited scarring, which tends to be confined to the adventitial dermis encompassing folliculosebaceous units. In contrast, NMPCA tends to be typified by a neutrophil-containing infiltrate in early disease, a mixed infiltrate in later disease, and marked scarring that extends beyond the perifollicular dermis and extensively involves the reticular (interfollicular) dermis. In late disease, when follicular density has been reduced and when the distinction between the adventitial dermis and the reticular dermis has been blurred, considerable overlap can be seen.

A criticism that has been levied against the LMPCA vs. NMPCA classification is that it represents a lumper's approach. Rather than holding out for new and better pathological criteria that permit precise distinction of traditional disease entities, the LMPCA vs. NMPCA method lumps certain time-honored categories. Utilizing this approach, LPP is not considered microscopically distinct from FFA, nor is tufted folliculitis considered microscopically distinct from folliculitis decalvans. Whether this criticism holds validity is a matter for debate. The criticism presumes that traditional categories of alopecia are all diseases *sui generis* and that an effort should be made to establish precise and distinctive histopathological definitions that safeguard them. While heretical to some, the opposing stance is that traditional clinical categories of alopecia may not be unique or histopathologically distinctive. Rather, the possibility should be considered that these clinical disease categories merely represent different and diverse clinical expressions of the same fundamental pathological (or disease) process. In short, if diseases such as LPP and FFA are histopathologically similar if not identical, perhaps an effort to assemble specific criteria that would permit their distinction might be destined to fail.

In the sections that follow, cicatricial alopecia will be broadly separated into LMPCA and NMPCA categories. Additionally, specific comments regarding the histopathology of specific traditional alopecic entities will be offered. For selected forms of alopecia, provisional categorization as mixed (rather than lymphocyte-mediated or neutrophil-mediated) cicatricial alopecia will be utilized. A brief overview of alopecia induced by lupus erythematosus, which is a lymphocyte-mediated disease but differs from other forms of LMPCA, is included.

Table 3.1 Histopathological distinction of LMPCA and NMPCA

	LMPCA	NMPCA
Infiltrate:	Rich in lymphocytes	Rich in neutrophils and histiocytes early, and rich in plasmacytes late
Sebaceous glands:	Loss affecting most follicles	Loss affecting most follicles
Compound follicles:	Fusion of two (rarely three) infundibula	Fusion of four or more infundibula
Fibrosis:	Limited to the adventitial dermis; concentric in areas of early involvement	Involves both the adventitial and reticular dermis jointly
Parafollicular granulomas:	Uncommon and few	Common and sometimes numerous

Lymphocyte-Mediated Primary Cicatricial Alopecias

LPP represents the prototypical form of cicatricial alopecia with an associated lymphocyte-rich infiltrate (1–3). Pseudopelade, as defined clinically by Brocq, represents its close differential diagnostic counterpart. For the histopathologist, the most common word combinations encountered on the requisition forms that accompany biopsy specimens submitted for evaluation of scarring alopecia include "LPP vs. pseudopelade" and "LPP vs. LE."

The term pseudopelade epitomizes the intractable difficulties that have been associated with the specific categorization of cicatricial alopecia. To many in the clinical realm, the designation pseudopelade holds vibrant import in reference to patients with multiple patches of alopecia, in which follicular markings have been lost, that is pelade-like (alopecia areata-like) in its distribution. In contrast, to many dermatopathologists, most notably the late Bernard Ackerman and many of his acolytes, the label pseudopelade has been utilized broadly as a generic equivalent for end-stage scarring alopecia.

FFA also represents a consensus member of the LMPCA group, and it has been clearly demonstrated that the separation of FFA from LPP is arbitrary (4,5). Additionally, we include central centrifugal cicatricial alopecia (CCCA) as a form of LMPCA (1), although the descriptions associated with that entity in some textbook references incorporate attributes that indicate that others are utilizing the designation differently. In some characterizations, CCCA has been utilized as a diagnosis for patients that we would interpret as suffering from a form of NMPCA.

Histopathologically, all patients with LMPCA are linked by the presence of a lymphocyte-rich infiltrate and scarring that tends to be accentuated in the perifollicular adventitial dermis. Although the infiltrate consists largely of lymphocytes, the designation LMPCA is not a connotation intended to convey that the process is strictly lymphocytic in nature. Admixed histocytes and eosinophils can be found in modest numbers, and occasionally small numbers of neutrophils are also included in the infiltrate.

The infiltrate tends to be exclusively perifollicular in distribution and band-like in configuration, although the character of the infiltrate is commonly disappointingly less lichenoid than conventional lichen planus (LP) (Fig. 3.2). While junctional vacuolar alteration and perijunctional necrotic keratinocytes are mainstays in the histopathology of conventional LP, often the degree of perifollicular keratinocytotoxicity associated with LPP, even in patients who suffer from concurrent epidermal LP, is muted. Exocytosis of many lymphocytes into the epithelium of follicular infundibulum and isthmus, without significant accompanying numbers of single necrotic keratinocytes, can be seen in some specimens. The perifollicular infiltrate varies considerably in density and distribution, and not uncommonly level sections are required to fully demonstrate the infiltrate in diagnostic biopsies. Although common sense suggests that the densest band-like infiltrate corresponds to early acute involvement and that a sparser infiltrate might be seen in later or waning disease, precise correlation of the density of the infiltrate with the time course of disease is generally not possible.

At times, there seems to be an inverse relationship between the lichenoid character of the

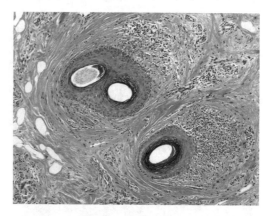

Fig. 3.2 At higher magnification, a lichenoid infiltrate surrounds one follicular structure. A compound follicle with two fused infundibula is apparent

perifollicular infiltrate and the degree of fibroplasia encountered with lymphocyte-mediated alopecia. In very early disease, an intense lichenoid infiltrate may be tightly wrapped around the folliculosebaceous unit and only modest perifollicular fibrosis is apparent. With disease progression, the degree of perifollicular fibroplasia becomes exaggerated and pushes the infiltrate away from follicular epithelium, often eventuating with morphology that is less compellingly lichenoid in character (Fig. 3.3). If level sections are examined, often a lichenoid infiltrate will be only focally detectable in biopsies from fully developed disease.

Perifollicular fibroplasia that is largely limited to the adventitial dermis also represents part and parcel of the histopathology of LMPCA. Early disease is typified by recent concentric fibroplasia that often assumes a slightly bluish hue in conventional sections due to the combination of fine collagen bundles and increased mucin. In later disease, coarser eosinophilic collagen is encountered. With late disease, coarse fibrosis or sclerosis of the entire follicular tract ensues after the follicular epithelium has been lost. A diminishment in the vascularity can also be seen in sclerotic follicular tracts.

From a histopathological standpoint, perifollicular fibroplasia is inversely linked to the prominence of sebaceous glands. In the normal situation, of course, sebaceous glands adorn

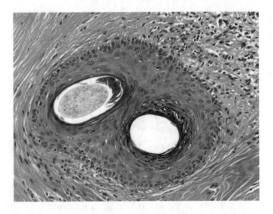

Fig. 3.3 At high magnification, only focal vacuolar alteration can be found within the compound follicular epithelium

virtually every follicular structure and perifollicular fibrosis is absent. In early LMPCA, loose concentric perifollicular fibroplasia is coupled with a reduction in the density of sebaceous glands. In late LMPCA, the degree of perifollicular fibrosis is typically marked and sebaceous glands are often not identifiable. The loss of sebaceous glands reflects the crucial role this gland plays in the pathogenesis of primary cicatricial alopecia (6).

Assessing the density of sebaceous glands at low magnification represents a useful step in an algorithmic approach to biopsy interpretation, especially when transverse sections are being evaluated. The uniform presence of sebaceous glands around all follicles in transverse sections favors interpretation as a nonscarring form of alopecia. If, in contrast, many or most follicles lack attached sebaceous glands and show encompassing concentric fibrosis, the diagnosis of cicatricial alopecia becomes certain. It is noteworthy that in the context of LMPCA, the loss of sebaceous glands may be uneven in biopsies obtained from recently diseased areas. Stated differently, partial preservation of sebaceous glands may be observed in biopsies obtained from areas of early cicatricial involvement.

Compound follicles, consisting of fused follicular infundibula that are encompassed by fibrosis, are not unique to any form of cicatricial alopecia. In LMPCA, compound follicles tend to be few in number and commonly only two (rarely three, exceptionally four) follicular infundibula are joined. If compound follicles representing the melding of five or more folliculosebaceous units are noted microscopically, then in all likelihood LMPCA does not represent the correct interpretation for the biopsy being evaluated.

Folliculosebaceous units tend not to rupture as a consequence of lymphocyte-mediated attack (Fig. 3.4), and thus extrusion of follicular contents into the dermis is limited. The salubrious effect of limited extrusion is that secondary inflammation elicited by keratinous debris is also limited. Because of this phenomenon, secondary granulomas are only occasionally found in association with LMPCA and tend to be small. A

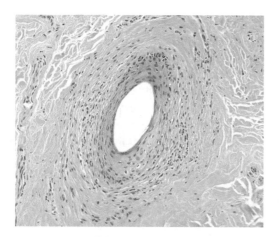

Fig. 3.4 Lymphocyte-mediated primary cicatricial alopecia (frontal fibrosing alopecia) at medium magnification. A sparse lymphocytic infiltrate that is minimally lichenoid is coupled with concentric perifollicular fibrosis that displays a myxoid quality. The encompassing reticular dermis is nonfibrotic

sporadic small sarcoidal collection of epithelioid histiocytes, sometimes encompassing an extrafollicular hair shaft, may be expected in this context. If an extensive secondary granulomatous infiltrate is encountered, the possibility of a diagnosis other than LMPCA should be strongly considered.

The clinical entities that present histopathologically as LMPCA include LPP, pseudopelade, FFA, and CCCA. LPP represents the prototypical form of LMPCA and the preceding paragraphs delineates its typical histopathology. In a small minority of cases of LPP, conventional LP can be found involving the superjacent epidermis. In comparing cases of LPP coupled with associated conventional LP to cases of LPP that lack associated epidermal involvement, we have been unable to identify any significant differences in the microscopical alterations afflicting folliculosebaceous units.

Pseudopelade is histopathologically indistinguishable from LPP. From the vantage of the dermatopathologist, distinctive clinical morphology represents the only reason for preservation of this diagnostic category.

FFA also shows great histopathological concordance with LPP. The case has been made that LPP and FFA represent the same disease (4,5).

Although in our experience this is a truism, a few subtle distinctions can be made. The number of involved folliculosebaceous units in FFA tends to be fewer in comparison to LPP. Although loss of sebaceous glands occurs as a secondary consequence of any cicatricial alopecia, reflecting the fact that scarring is centered on the follicular isthmus, where the sebaceous apparatus resides, the loss of sebaceous epithelium tends to be more conspicuous in biopsies of LPP. When the eyebrow involvement that commonly accompanies FFA is biopsied and examined microscopically, patchy scarring and partial preservation of sebaceous glands are particularly noteworthy findings.

As mentioned previously, CCCA represents the most controversial consideration in this listing. In our hands, the designation CCCA is defined clinically and its histopathology is similar if not identical to that of LPP and FFA (1). Descriptions of CCCA by other investigators that include references to clinical pustules indicate that the designation may be applied inconsistently in the clinical realm (7).

Lupus erythematosus (LE) represents a disease mediated by lymphocytes that often includes a component of alopecia as part of its course. LE is thus a common consideration in the differential diagnosis of LMPCA, although we believe the histopathology of LE is distinct from that of LPP and FFA. LE is typified histopathologically by a superficial and deep infiltrate that is often accompanied by mucin deposition in the reticular dermis. Vacuolar alteration of epidermal and adnexal epithelium tends to be more conspicuous in LE in comparison to LMPCA, and concentric fibrosis around infundibula tends not to be prominent. Compound follicles are few in number in LE. Utilizing the attributes discussed in the three preceding sentences, distinction of LE from NMPCA is possible in the vast majority of cases, particularly when the biopsy findings are coupled and correlated with the clinical context. For cases that are diagnostically challenging, utilization of CD123 immunostaining can be considered, as sizable collections of CD123-positive lymphocytes are common throughout the spectrum of LE and tend not to be identifiable in LP (8).

Neutrophil-Mediated Primary Cicatricial Alopecias

Folliculitis decalvans (FD) (Fig. 3.5) represents the prototypical form of cicatricial alopecia in which a neutrophil-rich infiltrate is prominent at certain disease phases (1,2). Although referred to as neutrophil-mediated, in part to maintain parallelism with LMPCA, it is important to recognize that it is not yet established that neutrophils play a primary or fundamental role in the pathogenesis of NMPCA, nor are neutrophils present in all biopsies obtained from patients with alopecia that is categorized as NMPCA. It remains conceivable that neutrophils are present in NMPCA as an epiphenomenon. That said, the identification of a neutrophil-rich infiltrate and/or evidence of neutrophilic folliculitis represent consistent findings, at least during certain disease phases, within the spectrum of NMPCA.

Cicatricial alopecia associated with a neutrophil-rich infiltrate may present with alterations that are situated relatively superficially or extremely deeply with respect to affected folliculosebaceous units. FD typically presents with superficial microscopical manifestations that are concentrated around the follicular infundibulum and isthmus, which collectively constitute the uppermost portion of the follicular structure. In contrast,

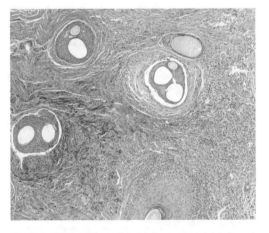

Fig. 3.5 Neutrophil-mediated primary cicatricial alopecia (folliculitis decalvans). The reticular dermis is diffusely fibrotic, holds a prominent infiltrate of mixed composition, and encompasses several compound follicles

the anomalies induced by dissecting cellulitis (discussed further in the section regarding mixed cicatricial alopecia that follows) typically encompass or fall deep to the follicular stem and bulb.

Infundibular pustules are identifiable clinically in patients with early or active FD, and the earliest histopathology associated with NMPCA is that of pustular folliculitis. Neutrophils can be found within follicular canals in concert with orthohyperkeratosis or parakeratosis, and attenuation or rupture of the infundibular epithelium may occur as a secondary consequence. The perifollicular infiltrate is mixed and includes varying numbers of neutrophils, histiocytes, lymphocytes, plasmacytes, and occasionally eosinophils. Acutely, perifollicular fibrosis may be inconspicuous, but secondary and circumferential perifollicular fibroplasia soon ensues as a consequence of infundibular rupture and is presumably fueled by extrusion of follicular contents.

The infiltrate in NMPCA varies considerably through the course of disease. Scalp biopsies from patients obtained relatively soon after the onset of alopecia demonstrate a granulocyte-rich infiltrate that is particularly prone to contain neutrophils. The degree of secondary perifollicular fibrosis varies but may be only modest. In contrast, biopsies obtained from patients with longstanding NMPCA include an infiltrate that contains many histiocytes and plasmacytes and generally display extensive secondary fibroplasia as well. The combination of a plasmacyte-rich infiltrate and exaggerated fibrosis, including both the adventitial dermis and the reticular dermis, is commonly present in association with late NMPCA and tends not to occur in LMPCA. When the combination is encountered in the evaluation of an alopecia biopsy, we believe it represents a strong clue to the diagnosis of NMPCA even in the absence of a neutrophilic infiltrate.

Folliculosebaceous units tend to rupture as a consequence of involvement by NMPCA, much as afflicted follicles tend to rupture as a consequence of conventional folliculitis, and thus extrusion of follicular contents into the dermis is expected. The consequence of follicular rupture is that secondary inflammation elicited by extruded keratinous debris is often marked.

Because of this phenomenon, secondary granulomas are commonly associated with NMPCA and at times are sizable. If an extensive secondary granulomatous infiltrate is encountered, the diagnosis is generally NMPCA and not LMPCA.

Follicular rupture and extrusion of follicular contents also fuel the marked secondary fibrosis that is common to NMPCA. Early in the course of disease, the degree of fibrosis may be modest and a concentric configuration much like that seen in LMPCA may be observed. In contrast, the degree of secondary fibrosis in later disease tends to be extremely exaggerated. With chronic involvement, secondary fibrosis extends beyond the perifollicular adventitial dermis and extensively involves the reticular (or interfollicular) dermis. At times, biopsies of late NMPCA will contain few follicles or residual follicular tracts and will merely display the configuration of a dermal scar. This is a reflection of extensive fibrosis that has extended far beyond the follicular adventitia.

As noted previously, compound follicles are not unique to any form of cicatricial alopecia. In the context of NMPCA, compound follicles tend to be conspicuous. Furthermore, the compound follicles associated with NMPCA commonly exhibit three, four, five, or more melded follicular infundibula (Fig. 3.6). If compound follicles representing the fusion of four or five folliculosebaceous units are noted microscopically, then a diagnosis of NMPCA is highly likely. If extremely high numbers of folliculosebaceous units (six or more) are fused, then a diagnosis of NMPCA is nearly certain.

FD represents the prototypical form of NMPCA and the preceding paragraphs delineate its typical histopathology. Tufted folliculitis, as defined clinically, represents a form of cicatricial typified by extreme compound follicle formation, and the compound follicles are manifested as tufts of preserved hairs within a backdrop of diffuse dermal scarring (9–12) (Fig. 3.7). Histopathologically, tufted folliculitis is identical to FD (9,10). The extreme compound follicle formation that is apparent clinically in patients with tufted folliculitis is also readily identifiable microscopically but does not provide a distinct means to separate tufted folliculitis from FD.

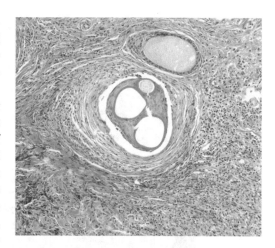

Fig. 3.6 At higher magnification, a compound follicle formed of three fused infundibula is apparent. Compound follicles formed of four or more fused infundibula are common to neutrophils-mediated alopecia and correspond to clinical tufts. In the surrounding fibrotic dermis, an infiltrate enriched in neutrophils and plasmacytes is appreciable

Erosive pustular dermatitis represents a form of scarring alopecia with associated folliculitis that often presents in elderly patients. The clinical lesions can be misconstrued as solar keratosis and squamous carcinoma. Some dermatopathologists take the stance that erosive pustular dermatitis does not represent a disease *sui generis*. Rather, some believe that the fibrosing inflammatory alterations that can be seen in patients with this clinical presentation are merely the epiphenomena of trauma. Suffice it to say that a mixed infiltrate, extensive perifollicular and reticular dermal fibrosis, and compound follicle formation can be seen in some patients with the clinical presentation of erosive pustular dermatitis. The histopathological spectrum of erosive pustular dermatitis may be nonspecific but overlaps with that of FD.

Mixed Cicatricial Alopecia

Although the breakdown of cicatricial alopecia into LMPCA and NMPCA provides a means to categorize the vast majority of patients, some traditional clinical diagnostic categories cannot be readily pigeonholed as they lack the qualities

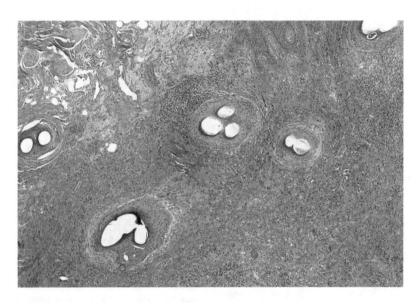

Fig. 3.7 Neutrophil-mediated primary cicatricial alopecia (clinically, tufted folliculitis). There are compound follicles within a diffusely fibrotic reticular dermis. The exaggerated (diffuse) dermal fibrosis is conspicuous in the lower right segment of the frame

shared by the various forms of lymphocyte-mediated and neutrophil-mediated alopecia. A provisional category of "mixed" scarring alopecia or cicatricial alopecia "not otherwise specified" is maintained to include patients with such involvement (2). Patients with cicatricial alopecia associated with acneiform follicular hyperkeratosis are included in this spectrum. Dissecting cellulitis and acne keloidalis represent examples of scarring diseases that are not readily classifiable as either LMPCA or NMPCA.

In some patients, the pathological spectrum of dissecting cellulitis overlaps extensively with FD. Dissecting cellulitis is manifested histopathologically with marked reduction in follicular density; a mixed infiltrate that includes neutrophils, histiocytes, lymphocytes, and plasmacytes; and an extensive coarse fibrosis that involves both the perifollicular adventitial dermis and the interfollicular dermis (Fig. 3.8). Compound follicles may be seen but are not necessarily conspicuous. Deep sinus tract formation can be seen. The clinical presentation of dissecting cellulitis patients with deeply situated, boggy plaques parallels what is observed microscopically in that the scarring associated with the disorder tends to span the full reticular dermis and also extensively replaces

the subcutis that falls deep to the follicular bulb and stem. In comparison to FD, the secondary scarring elicited by dissecting cellulitis tends to be both more extensive and more deeply situated. At times, the deep scarring associated with dissecting cellulitis will extend subjacent to areas in which follicular density remains normal. This corresponds clinically to an area in which a boggy quality has developed but in which clinical alopecia has not yet ensued.

Similarly, biopsies obtained from the scalps of patients with acne keloidalis show varied histopathology. The common theme is marked dermal fibrosis that encompasses distorted folliculosebaceous units. Many of the affected follicles show infundibular plugging by compact orthohyperkeratosis or by compact parakeratosis. Plugged follicles often rupture, and the consequent extrusion of follicular contents fuels both scarring and secondary inflammation. The associated secondary infiltrate can vary greatly in its composition. Most commonly, the infiltrate is granulomatous or rich in plasmacytes. Lymphocytes and neutrophils may be present concurrently in varying numbers. Acne keloidalis represents a disease that is uncommonly biopsied. As the disease can typically be defined based upon clinical

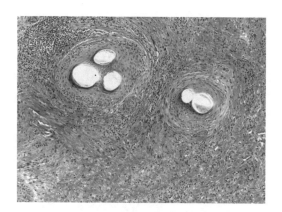

Fig. 3.8 At higher magnification, compound follicles are encompassed by a diffusely fibrotic dermis. Neutrophils are inconspicuous in the dermal infiltrate at this late phase of disease

morphology, histopathological examination is not required for a specific diagnosis to be rendered.

An ongoing problem inherent to the histopathological evaluation of cicatricial alopecia is the assessment of biopsies from patients with late or "end-stage" disease that is not readily pigeonholed. Such biopsies often include few viable follicles upon which to base meaningful conclusions. Little infiltrate may remain in a sample of late alopecia, and thus a key means to permit distinction of LMPCA from NMPCA may be ineffectual in this context. In particular, specimens obtained from end-stage NMPCA with a minimal remaining chronic infiltrate may be misinterpreted and misclassified as examples of LMPCA. It is crucial to remember that little can be gained through the analysis of end-stage alopecia. If such patients have remaining active alopecia, such areas should preferentially be utilized as the source of biopsy material and as the basis for clinical and histopathological classification.

References

1. Mirmirani P, Willey A, Headington JT, et al. Primary cicatricial alopecia: histopathologic findings do not distinguish clinical variants. J Am Acad Dermatol. 2005;52:637–43.
2. Stefanato CM. Histopathology of alopecia: a clinicopathological approach to diagnosis. Histopathology. 2010;56:24–38.
3. Sullivan JR, Kossard S. Acquired scalp alopecia: a review. Australas J Dermatol. 1998;39:207–19; 220–21.
4. Kossard S, Lee MS, Wilkinson B. Postmenopausal frontal fibrosing alopecia: a frontal variant of lichen planopilaris. J Am Acad Dermatol. 1997;36:59–66.
5. Kossard S. Postmenopausal frontal fibrosing alopecia. Scarring alopecia in a pattern distribution. Arch Dermatol. 1994;130:770–4.
6. Stenn, Karnik P. Lipids to the top of hair biology. J Invest Dermatol. 2010;130:1205–7.
7. Sperling LC. Scarring alopecia and the dermatopathologist. J Cutan Pathol. 2001;28:333–42.
8. Tomasini D, Mentzel T, Hantschke M, et al. Plasmacytoid dendritic cells: an overview of their presence and distribution in different inflammatory skin diseases, with special emphasis on Jessner's lymphocytic infiltrate of the skin and cutaneous lupus erythematosus. J Cutan Pathol. 2010;37:1132–9.
9. Powell JJ, Dawber RP, Gatter K. Folliculitis decalvans including tufted folliculitis: clinical, histological and therapeutic findings. Br J Dermatol. 1999; 140(2):328–33.
10. Annessi G. Tufted folliculitis of the scalp: a distinctive clinicohistological variant of folliculitis decalvans. Br J Dermatol. 1998;138:799–805.
11. Pujol RM, García-Patos V, Ravella-Mateu A, et al. Tufted hair folliculitis: a specific disease? Br J Dermatol. 1994;130:259–60.
12. Tong AK, Baden HP. Tufted hair folliculitis. J Am Acad Dermatol. 1989;21:1096–99.

Medical Management

4

Vera Price and Paradi Mirmirani

The management of cicatricial alopecia will change as our understanding of the molecular pathogenesis increases. With this increased knowledge, it is likely that the classification will be revised and offer new therapeutic strategies.

A scalp biopsy is the essential first step in assessing a patient with cicatricial alopecia (see Chap. 2). If time is limited, a thorough evaluation need not be completed on the first visit. Most important, take the scalp biopsy on the first visit and complete the evaluation at the next visit.

Choice of Treatment

The important features of the dermatopathology report are described in Chap. 3. Based on the predominant cellular infiltrate, histopathologic findings can separate the predominantly lymphocytic group and the predominantly neutrophilic group. Although this does not distinguish the various clinical forms, the nature of the inflammatory filtrate provides a practical guide for selecting treatments. Medical treatment options are broadly grouped into treatments for lymphocytic and for neutrophilic/plasmacytic cicatricial alopecia. Recent molecular research has shown that peroxisome proliferator-activated receptor gamma (PPAR-gamma) expression is significantly decreased in lichen planopilaris. For this reason, PPAR gamma agonists or glitazones are listed as a new treatment option for lichen planopilaris.

Counseling and Setting Expectations

Current treatments are not perfect, but the distress and suffering of patients are real, so that careful listening, an understanding approach, and an informed discussion about cicatricial alopecia all go far in helping the patient.

Explain the good news about cicatricial alopecia: it has no effect on general health, it occurs in otherwise healthy people, it is not contagious, and not hereditary. Nevertheless, the patient's distress is understandable and needs to be validated. Most patients have never heard of cicatricial alopecia and a brief explanation is helpful: why are these disorders called "cicatricial or scarring", and why is the hair loss permanent? Connect the patient to sources of sound information such as the Cicatricial Alopecia Research Foundation (CARF) (www.carfintl.org).

Prior to counseling the patient on treatment options, it is essential to explain that the goal of treatment is to (a) alleviate the symptoms and clinical signs and (b) retard or slow the progression of the disease. The patient should also understand that regrowth of hair is not possible and activity may recur after months or years. With this understanding, the clinician and the patient can work together to evaluate the efficacy of treatments. The therapeutic plan is generally based on the extent of the inflammatory infiltrate on biopsy (sparse, moderate, dense) and on clinical assessment of the disease.

V. Price and P. Mirmirani (eds.), *Cicatricial Alopecia: An Approach to Diagnosis and Management*,
DOI 10.1007/978-1-4419-8399-2_4, © Springer Science+Business Media, LLC 2011

Components of the clinical assessment include:

1. Symptoms (itching, pain, burning)
2. Clinical signs (perifollicular erythema, perifollicular scale, erythema, pustules, crusting, pull test: anagen/total)
3. Spreading of hair loss (determined by patient self-report, review of photographs, clinical exam, and measurements if practical)

These three specific outcome measures are evaluated and recorded approximately every 3 months on a flow chart. The vast array of treatments for cicatricial alopecia described in the literature needs to be evaluated in this context. The treatment guidelines listed below are not meant to be exhaustive, but instead reflect the practices of the authors at this time. Although not specific for the treatment of cicatricial alopecia, we sometimes add minoxidil solution or Rogaine foam to maximize the growth of unaffected hair.

If the outcome measures show improvement, the systemic agents are continued for 6 to 12 months. On the other hand, if there is no improvement after 3 months, then an alternative systemic drug is considered. With improvement in the outcome measures, this drug is continued for 6 to 12 months. Specific therapeutic options, combinations, and challenges are discussed in the chapters for the various disorders.

Treatment of Predominantly Lymphocytic Cicatricial Alopecia

Treatment approaches for the lymphocytic group are immunomodulating agents and PPAR-gamma agonists.
Oral:
1st tier: hydroxychloroquine 200 mg twice daily for 6–12 months, or doxycycline 100 mg twice daily for 6–12 months, or
2nd tier: mycophenolate mofetil 0.5 gm twice daily for first month, then 1 gm twice daily for 5 months, or cyclosporine 3–5 mg/kg per day or 300 mg/day for 3–5 months, or

3rd tier: pioglitazone 15 mg daily or rosiglitazone 4 mg daily for 3–6 months, particularly for lichen planopilaris.

Topical: high potency corticosteroids, tacrolimus or pimecrolimus
> *Note:* To make topical tacrolimus suitable for the scalp, we often prescribe compounded tacrolimus 0.1% in Cetaphil® lotion and request a pointed tip applicator.

Derma-Smoothe/FS scalp oil
Anti-seborrheic shampoos

Intralesional: Injection of triamcinolone acetonide 10 mg/cc to inflamed, symptomatic sites

Treatment of Predominantly Neutrophilic/Plasmacytic Cicatricial Alopecia

Treatment approach for the neutrophilic group is antimicrobial agents.

Culture scalp pustules whenever they are present and obtain sensitivities.

Select oral microbials based on the predominant pathogens and resistance patterns in a given community. If no pustules are present, lift up a site of scalp crusting and culture underlying skin, or culture a small deep scalp biopsy, or alternatively culture hair bulbs (obtained in a pull test).

For *staphylocccus aureus*

Oral. Cephalexin 500 mg 4 times daily for 10 weeks with oral rifampin 600 mg every morning for 10 days. May substitute: clindamycin 300 mg twice daily, or ciprofloxacin 750 mg twice daily, or doxycycline 100 mg twice daily, all given for 10 weeks and with rifampin 600 mg every morning for 10 days; or sulfamethoxazole-trimethoprim DS twice daily for 10 weeks.

Topical. Clindamycin phosphate topical solution 1%, or clindamycin phosphate topical gel 1%, dapsone gel 5%, mupirocin ointment or cream, and Derma-Smoothe/FS scalp oil (sometimes soothing, sometimes not tolerated), antiseborrheic shampoos.

Intralesional. Injection of triamcinolone acetonide 10 mg/cc to inflamed, symptomatic sites

Culture nostrils. If *staph* carrier, apply topical mupirocin ointment to nostrils daily for 1 week, then once per month.

For dissecting cellulitis. Culture often does not grow a pathogen. Isotretinoin is helpful in some patients. Starting dose must be small: 10–20 mg per day for 6–12 months.

For infliximab, adalimumab, etanercept in dissecting cellulitis, see "Dissecting cellulitis" in Chap. 8.

For folliculitis keloidalis: for early mild disease: class 1 or class 2 topical corticosteroids with or without topical antibiotics; for papules and nodules: intralesional triamcinolone acetonide (10 mg/ml) every 4–6 weeks, along with topical antibiotics, or oral antibiotics such as tetracycline, doxycycline, minocycline; for advanced disease, excisional surgery may be necessary.

Laboratory Workup and Side Effects of Systemic Drugs

Hydroxychloroquine

An ophthalmologic exam including a retinal exam is done at the outset in all patients along with a CBC and liver function tests. The eye exam is repeated after an interval suggested by the ophthalmologist (usually 6–12 months) and the blood tests are not repeated if normal at the start. In addition, patients of African ancestry are tested for glucose-6-phosphate dehydrogenase deficiency. The most common side effects are gastrointestinal symptoms. Patients with glucose-6-phopsphate dehydrogenase deficiency should not take this medication.

Doxycycline

No pretreatment laboratory workup is required. The most common side effects include gastrointestinal symptoms, photosensitivity, headache, and candidiasis. An option for women with a history of vaginal candidiasis is to give fluconazole 150 mg p.o. once every month.

Mycophenolate Mofetil

Baseline CBC and liver function tests are obtained at the outset. The tests are repeated again after 4 weeks and every 12 weeks thereafter. The most common adverse events are gastrointestinal disturbances, peripheral edema, fatigue, and opportunistic infection (herpes zoster).

Cyclosporine

Baseline tests include blood pressure, serum creatinine (checked twice), CBC, liver function tests, BUN, and urinalysis. Follow-up monitoring of blood pressure, serum creatinine, CBC, liver function tests are performed at 2 weeks, 4 weeks, and monthly thereafter. When cyclosporine is used as monotherapy, the most common side effects include elevated creatinine (renal dysfunction), hypertension, hypertrichosis, flu-like symptoms, and gastrointestinal disturbances.

Pioglitazone/Rosiglitazone

Recently, we have had success treating patients with LPP with PPAR-gamma agonists or glitazones, which are medications that are widely used and FDA-approved for the treatment of type 2 diabetes mellitus. Pioglitazone and rosiglitazone are the currently available glitazones in the United States.

The glitazones are new to the roster of systemic treatments for the predominantly lymphocytic cicatricial alopecias, particularly for lichen planopilaris, and the duration of treatment is not known. Since these medications lower blood glucose by improving insulin sensitivity, they can be safely used in nondiabetic patients. Baseline weight, CBC, and liver function tests are obtained prior to treatment. Weight and blood pressure are monitored monthly, and CBC and liver function tests are repeated every 12 weeks. The main side effects of these medications include: dosage-dependent fluid retention and secondary peripheral edema and weight gain as a result of renal sodium reabsorption. This fluid retention may pose a cardiovascular risk in patients predisposed to congestive heart failure. Hypoglycemia does not occur in nondiabetics. Pioglitazone induces cytochrome P450 and raises the possibility of drug interactions, such as with oral contraceptives (lowering efficacy). When compared to other oral medications used for treatment of LPP and other cicatricial alopecias, the glitazones have an acceptable side effect and safety profile.

Rifampin

Rifampin is indispensable for the treatment of both methicillin-resistant *staphylococcus aureus* and *streptococcus pyogenes* when combination therapy is warranted. However, resistance develops quickly when this agent is used as monotherapy. Rifampin is also a potent inducer of the cytochrome P-450 oxidative system and careful review of the patient's current medications is needed to rule out any clinically significant drug interactions such as with oral contraceptives and coumadin (lowering efficacy).

Sulfamethoxazole Trimethoprim DS

Ask if the patient has a history of kidney or liver disease. Patients with glucose-6-phopsphate dehydrogenase deficiency should not take this medication. The most common side effects include gastrointestinal symptoms and photosensitivity.

Confounding Factors in Managing Cicatricial Alopecias

- After laying out a systematic approach to the management of the patient with cicatricial alopecia, we have to add that in a few patients

the cicatricial alopecia does not respond as hoped and proves to be challenging.

- Clinical and histologic findings may change over time: a neutrophilic cicatricial alopecia may become lymphocytic and the failure to respond to treatment indicates the need for a rebiopsy that will demonstrate this change.
- At other times, the histology may not correlate with response to treatment: the predominant infiltrate may be neutrophilic, but the patient does not respond to antimicrobials and does respond to an immunomodulating drug. Other times, a predominantly lymphocytic inflammation responds to an antimicrobial agent and not to an immunomodulating drug.
- The clinician sometimes faces a dilemma regarding which treatment to select: immunomodulating or antimicrobial agent?
- If a neutrophilic cicatricial alopecia is notably difficult to control, take repeated cultures. Suspect an anaerobic bacterial presence. Question the patient about household pets (dogs), the patient's occupation, and work surroundings.
- Another difficulty is that many patients present with late-stage disease, which is problematic for both diagnosis and treatment. Only acute phase lesions are diagnostic, and clinical and histologic assessment must be made on early stages. Historically, end-stage disease has been a major pitfall in managing cicatricial alopecia and has added to the nosologic and therapeutic challenge these disorders present.

Suggested Reading

Alikahn A, Lynch PJ, Eisen DB. Hidradenitis suppurativa: a comprehensive review. J Am Acad Dermatol. 2009;60:539–61.

Buell C, Koo J. Long-term safety of mycophenolate mofetil and cyclosporine: a review. J Drugs Dermatol. 2008;7:741–8.

Chiang C, Sah D, Cho BK et al. Hydroxychloroquine and lichen planopilaris: efficacy and introduction of Lichen Planopilaris Activity Index scoring system. J Am Acad Dermatol. 2010; 62:387–92.

Cho BK, Sah D, Chwalek J, et al. Efficacy and safety of mycophenolate mofetil for lichen planopilaris. J Am Acad Dermatol. 2010;62:393–7.

Grant A, Gonzalez T, Montgomery MO. Infliximab therapy for patients with moderate to severe hidradenitis suppurativa: a randomized, double-blind, placebo-controlled crossover trial. J Am Acad Dermatol. 2010;62:205–17.

Harries MJ, Sinclair RD, Macdonald-Hull S, et al. Management of primary cicatricial alopecias: Options for treatment. Br J Dermatol. 2008;159:1–22.

Lebwohl B, Sapadin AN. Infliximab for the treatment of hidradenitis suppurativa. J Am Acad Dermatol. 2003;49:S275–6.

Mekkes JR, Bos JD. Long-term efficacy of a single course of infliximab in hidradenitis suppurativa. Br J Dermatol. 2008;158:370–4.

Mirmirani P, Karnik P. Lichen planopilaris treated with a peroxisome proliferator-activated receptor gamma agonist. Arch Dermatol. 2009;145:1363–6.

Price VH. The medical treatment of cicatricial alopecia. Semin Cutan Med Surg. 2006;25:56–9.

Ross EK, Tan E, Shapiro J. Update on primary cicatricial alopecias. J Am Acad Dermatol. 2005;53: 1–37.

Tan E, Martinka M, Ball N, et al. Primary cicatricial alopecias: clinicopathology of 112 cases. 2004;50: 25–32.

Trehan, M. The use of antimalarials in dermatology. J Dermatol Treat. 2000;11:185–94.

Whiting DA. Cicatricial alopecia: clinico-pathological findings and treatment. Clin Dermatol. 2001;19: 211–25.

Mechanisms and Current Research

5

Vera Price and Paradi Mirmirani

Overview

Until recently, primary cicatricial alopecias had received little attention in the clinical and research realm. With the dramatic increases in our knowledge of basic hair biology, new and powerful tools have become available to study these rare disorders in ways that were previously not possible. As we have moved from traditional clinical studies and histopathology to molecular biology, new paradigms regarding the pathophysiology of cicatricial alopecia have been developed. However, after clarifying many previously unanswered questions, we are faced with a series of new and unanswered ones. By the time this publication is completed, new information will be available, and we encourage the reader to stay tuned and engaged as research in cicatricial alopecia continues to unfold.

Animal Models and the Sebotrophic Hypothesis

Mouse models with mutations of genes expressed in the mouse sebaceous gland, specifically the asebia mouse (stearyl-coenzyme A desaturase gene) and defolliculated (gasdermin 3-a transcription factor), have a clinical and histologic picture similar to cicatricial alopecia seen in humans. This work was the first to suggest that the sebaceous gland may be central to the pathogenesis of cicatricial alopecias. The sebotrophic hypothesis put forth the notion that the desquamation of the inner root sheath is dependent on the normal function of the sebum and that the absence of the normal sebaceous gland leads to obstructed outflow of the hair shaft. Subsequently, there is inflammation and eventual destruction of the follicle. Although the sebaceous gland plays a central role, the problem could be proximal or distal to this gland, leaving room for the possibility that environment, toxins, infection, and other triggers may play an initial role.

Studies reviewing the histopathology of cicatricial alopecias have consistently found loss of sebaceous glands in the affected tissue. In addition, biopsies of clinically unaffected scalp in patients with lichen planopilaris have shown early sebaceous gland atrophy. The sebaceous gland thus became an active target for study.

Stem Cells and Immunology

The failure of affected follicles to regrow in primary cicatricial alopecia is thought to be due to destructive inflammatory changes at the level of the insertion of the arrector pili muscle into the region of the follicular bulge. This is the location of the slow cycling hair follicle stem cells that are capable of initiating follicular renewal at the end of the normal resting phase of the hair cycle. Studies have shown that the hair follicle stem cells and not the epidermal stem cells are injured in the primary cicatricial alopecias. However, it has been unclear whether the stem cells are the primary target in the disease or innocent bystanders that are destroyed as a result of the inflammatory insult.

V. Price and P. Mirmirani (eds.), *Cicatricial Alopecia: An Approach to Diagnosis and Management*, DOI 10.1007/978-1-4419-8399-2_5, © Springer Science+Business Media, LLC 2011

Prior studies have found that the human hair follicle appears to have immune privilege with major histocompatibility complex (MHC) class I negativity and an immunosuppressive cytokine milieu. In normal anagen hair, macrophages are located primarily in the perifollicular connective tissue sheath and are virtually absent from the hair follicle epithelium. It has been suggested that the physiologic role of macrophages may be to scavenge excess basement membrane collagen during hair follicle regression and to eliminate abnormal or malfunctioning hair follicles by "programmed organ deletion". A collapse of immune privilege may lead to the elimination of hair follicles in cicatricial alopecia; this may occur under pathologic circumstances and with loss of the important "no danger" signal CD200.

Lipid Metabolic Pathways and Peroxisomes

More recent work suggests that one type of primary cicatricial alopecia, specifically lichen planopilaris, is a lipid metabolic disorder caused by a down-regulation of the peroxisome proliferator-activated receptor gamma (PPAR-gamma). Peroxisomes are single membrane bound, ubiquitous, subcellular organelles catalyzing a number of indispensable functions in the cell including lipid metabolism and the decomposition of harmful hydrogen peroxide. The importance of peroxisomes in humans is stressed by the existence of an ever expanding, diverse, and often fatal group of inherited peroxisomal biogenesis disorders (PBDs). Several cutaneous manifestations of PBDs have been reported and it is intriguing to note that patients with the peroxisomal disorder, X-linked dominant or recessive CDP (XCDP2), display epidermal hyperkeratosis and follicular plugging with cicatricial alopecia. The hypothesis that LPP is an acquired peroxisome biogenesis disorder that is localized to the scalp pilosebaceous unit was a novel concept that was based on results from comparative gene-expression profiling as well as a number of other subsequent supportive studies.

Microarray experiments with scalp biopsies from patients with lichen planopilaris compared affected and unaffected scalp, as well as scalp biopsies from control patients without LPP. These studies revealed major biological pathways that were upregulated, including inflammatory and cell death pathways, whereas lipid metabolic and hair follicle cycling and development were downregulated. Interestingly, the metabolic changes were noted in both affected and unaffected scalp biopsies in LPP, whereas the inflammatory changes were marked in affected scalp biopsies only. A bioinformatics program, Ingenuity Pathways Analysis, was used to further study the inflammatory pathways identified in the microarray experiments. Most of the upregulated inflammatory networks were seen in affected but not in unaffected LPP tissue, nor in controls, suggesting that although components of the inflammatory cascade such as cytokines, chemokines, and adhesion receptors are important in disease progression, they may not represent the primary events in the pathogenesis of LPP.

The most significant down-regulated biologic pathways in the affected and unaffected LPP scalp biopsies involved fatty acid metabolism, fatty acid desaturation, and cholesterol biosynthesis. Another group of genes that were downregulated in affected and unaffected LPP were those required for peroxisome biogenesis. It was hypothesized that the differentially expressed genes in LPP might be regulated by a common transcription factor or master regulator. Bioinformatics analysis revealed PPAR response elements on all down-regulated genes. Further experiments including PCR and cell culture analysis pointed toward a key role for PPAR-gamma in the pathogenesis of LPP. A mouse model with a targeted hair follicle stem cell deletion of PPAR-gamma demonstrated many of the gene expression and histologic findings of LPP (Fig. 5.1).

Accumulating evidence in the literature suggests that PPAR-gamma expression may be affected by environmental response genes. Intriguingly, the aryl hydrocarbon receptor that was found to be upregulated in microarray analysis of LPP patients is known to suppress PPAR-gamma in response to dioxin-like substances.

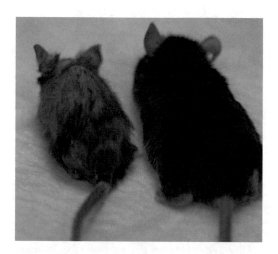

Fig. 5.1 Targeted disruption of PPAR- gamma in stem cells of the hair follicle bulge in mice resulted in scarring alopecia with loss of follicular markings and erythema. On the left, knockout mouse is smaller compared to normal littermate on the right. In the knockout mice, hair loss occurred in patchy areas and the mice exhibited severe scratching behavior

Based on this work, a new model of the pathogenesis of cicatricial alopecia has been developed (Fig. 5.2). External, environmental, and/or genetic triggers may lead to localized peroxisomal dysfunction, and result in abnormal lipid homeostasis and lipid accumulation, causing tissue damage (lipotoxicity) of the pilosebaceous unit. This tissue damage then triggers chemokine/cytokine expression, recruits lymphocytes, and macrophages, and activates a lipid-mediated programmed cell death (lipoapoptosis) and results in permanent hair loss in LPP. These pathways may be perturbed in the other types of primary cicatricial alopecia as well.

Other studies have also pointed to the importance of the sebaceous gland and normal lipid pathways in maintaining a healthy hair follicle. In 2007, a serendipitous observation was noted in a mammary gland-specific knockout mouse. The mice themselves had no visible changes or specific phenotype, but nursing pups of the mutant mice developed alopecia induced by toxic oxidized lipids carried in the mothers' milk. Once the pups were weaned, their hair loss was reversed. This striking observation suggests the vital role of lipid homeostasis in normal hair follicles. More recently, cholesterol metabolism has been shown to affect hair biology in a mouse model with up-regulated cholesterol synthesis due to the knockout of Insig proteins (inhibitors of 3-hydroxy-3 methylglutaryl coenzyme A reductase, the rate limiting enzyme of cholesterol biosynthesis). There appears to be a clear link between altered lipid metabolism and a toxic effect on the hair follicle. The exact pathways by which follicular inflammation and fibrosis occur have not been fully worked out. It may be that various upstream triggers or insults lead to a final common pathway of inflammation or fibrosis. Opportunities for pharmacologic intervention in primary cicatricial alopecias may be increased once the upstream triggers as well as the downstream inflammatory responses can be adequately identified.

Future Areas of Research and Unanswered Questions/ Controversies

Can a molecular classification of primary cicatricial alopecias be developed? Although our current classification of primary cicatricial alopecias is based on histopathologic characteristics, it is clear that this methodology has its limits in separating the different clinical patterns seen in patients. We have kept the histopathologic classification in this text as it serves as a familiar and convenient starting point when discussing these disorders. However, as we learn more about the molecular pathways in primary cicatricial alopecia, we will be able to better classify these disorders and also identify more targeted treatments. An initial step in such a molecular classification may be to separate those disorders in which there is abnormal lipid/metabolic metabolism due to decreased PPAR-gamma expression. Preliminary data suggests that the predominantly lymphocytic disorders lichen planopilaris, frontal fibrosing alopecia, and pseudopelade have disordered PPAR-gamma function. Although PPAR gamma expression is not decreased in central centrifugal cicatricial alopecia (CCCA), a co-activator of PPAR-gamma is decreased. The predominantly neutrophilic primary cicatricial alopecias require further molecular study.

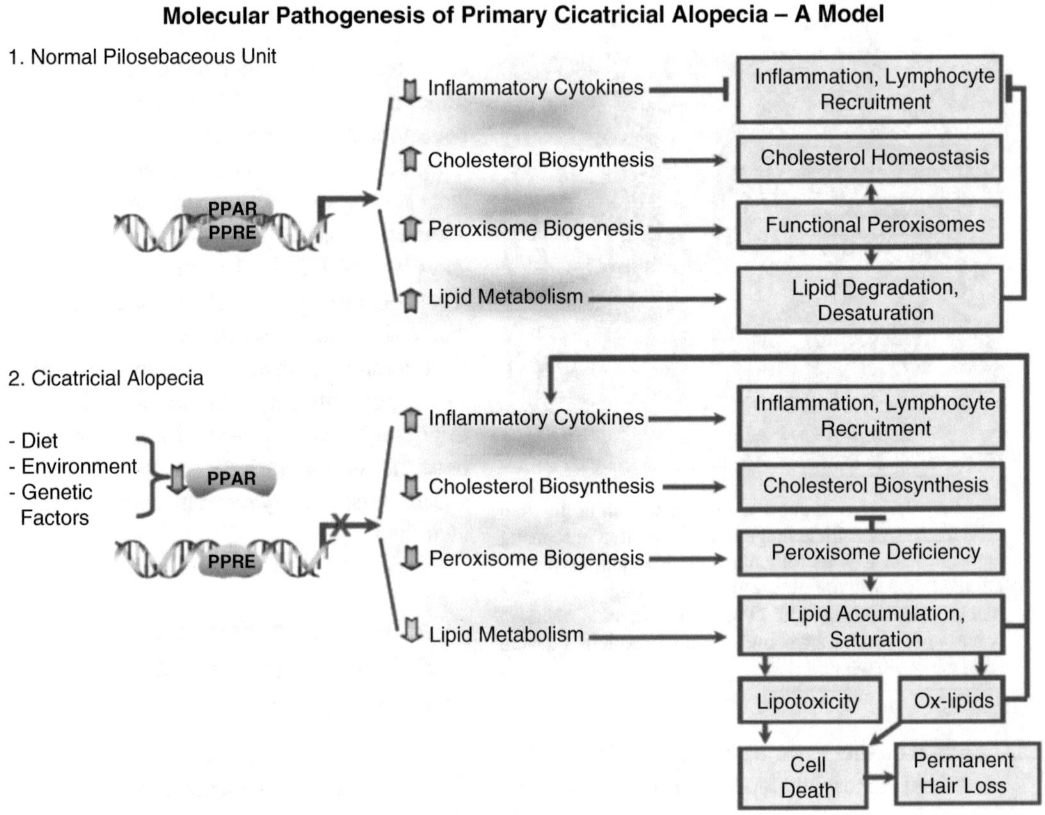

Molecular Pathogenesis of Primary Cicatricial Alopecia – A Model

1. Normal Pilosebaceous Unit

2. Cicatricial Alopecia

- Diet
- Environment
- Genetic
  Factors

Fig. 5.2 A new model of the pathogenesis of lichen planopilaris: External, environmental and/or genetic triggers may lead to localized peroxisomal dysfunction, and result in abnormal lipid homeostasis and lipid accumulation, causing tissue damage (lipotoxicity) of the pilosebaceous unit. This tissue damage then triggers chemokine/cytokine expression, recruits lymphocytes and macrophages and activates a lipid-mediated programmed cell death (lipoapoptosis) and results in permanent hair loss in LPP

Chronic cutaneous lupus erythematosus (CCLE) belongs to the autoimmune spectrum of lupus erythematosus, which is considered a primary inflammatory disorder. To our knowledge, the pathogenesis of CCLE has not been linked to disturbed PPAR-gamma. Additionally, since the inflammatory response in CCLE is not specifically directed at the folliculosebaceous unit, but is also superficial, deep, peri-vascular, and peri-appendageal (peri-eccrine), this disorder should be separated from other primary cicatricial alopecias.

Folliculitis keloidalis and dissecting cellulitis appear to result from mechanical rupture of the hair follicle with the released sebaceous material and keratin causing intense granulomatous inflammation. Although these two disorders and other primary cicatricial alopecias share some features including loss of normal sebaceous glands, the initial trigger leading to sebaceous gland dysfunction is likely distinct.

Suggested Reading

Evers B, Farooqi MS, Shelton JM, et al. Hair growth defects in Insig-deficient mice caused by cholesterol precursor accumulation and reversed by simvastatin. J Invest Dermatol. 2010;130:1237–48.

Karnik P, Tekeste Z, McCormick TS, et al. Hair follicle stem cell-specific PPARgamma deletion causes scarring alopecia. J Invest Dermatol. 2009;129:1243–57.

Stenn K, Karnik P. Lipids to the top of hair biology. J Invest Dermatol. 2010;130:1205–7.

Wan Y, Saghatelian A, Chong L, et al. Maternal PPAR gamma protects nursing neonates by suppressing the production of inflammatory milk. Genes Dev. 2007;21:1895–1908.

Predominantly Lymphocytic Group

6

Vera Price and Paradi Mirmirani

In this chapter, lichen planopilaris, Graham Little syndrome, frontal fibrosing alopecia (FFA), pseudopelade (Brocq), and central centrifugal cicatricial alopecia are described. Two additional entities that are not primary cicatricial alopecias are included, namely chronic cutaneous lupus erythematosus (CCLE) and keratosis follicularis spinulosa decalvans (KFSD) because they are important to recognize and differentiate.

The presentation is practical and detailed, and reflects our approach to the cicatricial alopecias. At the beginning of each chapter, a clinical scenario of one of our patients is described, and we highlight features of the history and exam that are clues to the diagnosis and list biopsy findings that support the diagnosis. A discussion of the disease follows with illustrative figures. Each chapter concludes with take-away pearls that highlight useful information for the clinician. Finally, suggested reading is listed but is not intended to be an exhaustive list of references.

Lichen Planopilaris

Clinical Scenario

A 47-year-old Caucasian woman seeks care for the sudden onset of scalp irritation, severe itching and pain, and rapid patchy hair loss. The patient has no other significant medical problems; she takes no prescription medications. On exam, she has exceptionally thick hair. On closer exam after parting the hair in sections, there are scattered 2–3 cm patches of hair loss throughout the scalp with absent follicular markings. At the margins of the patches, there is perifollicular scaling and perifollicular erythema (Fig. 6.1). A pull test at the margin is positive for anagen hair. Scalp biopsy is taken from the site of the anagen positive pull test (but could have been taken from any site along the active border). At the initial visit, her clinical parameters (symptoms, signs, progression of her hair loss) are documented on the standardized cicatricial alopecia flow chart (Table 6.1).

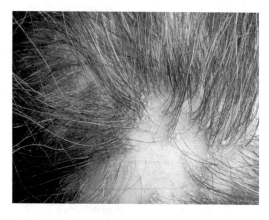

Fig. 6.1 LPP with perifollicular erythema, perifollicular scaling, and diminished follicular ostia

V. Price and P. Mirmirani (eds.), *Cicatricial Alopecia: An Approach to Diagnosis and Management*, DOI 10.1007/978-1-4419-8399-2_6, © Springer Science+Business Media, LLC 2011

Table 6.1 Example of the standardized flow chart of LPP patient, described in the Clinical scenario, at baseline and after 3 months of treatment with hydroxychloroquine

Name		Diagnosis	Lichen planopilaris		
Date of visit	12/7/2009	3/7/2010			
LPPAI (see Table 6.2)	9.33	2.33			
A Pruritus	++	+/–			
B Pain	++	+/–			
C Burning	+/–	–			
D Erythema	++	+/–			
E Perifollicular erythema	++	+			
F Perifollicular scale	+	+			
* Crusting	–	–			
* Pustules	–	–			
Pull test: Anagen hairs/Total hairs	2/4	0/3			
Spreading	Yes	No			
Dimensions/Extent	Scattered 2–3 cm patches throughout the scalp	Scattered 2–3 cm patches throughout the scalp			
* Loss follicular of markings	+	+			
* Tufting	+	+			
* Telangiectasia	–	–			
* Atrophy	–	–			
* Pigment change	–	–			
* Other skin, nail, mucous membrane	–	–			
Labs CBC	Ordered	Normal			
Date of visit	12/7/2009	3/7/2010			
AST/ALT/Alk Phos	Ordered	Normal			
G6PD	–	–			
Eye exam	Ordered	Normal			
BUN/CR	–	–			
Blood Pressure	–	–			
Culture & Sensitivities	–	–			
Treatment/Comments	If labs and eye exam normal, start hydroxy-chloroquine 200 mg BID	Continue hydroxychloroquine 200 mg BID			
Biopsy	11/2009				
Photographs	Yes				
F/U visit	3 months	3 months			

The LPPAI calculation is explained in Table 6.2

Scale A–F: negative =–, questionable or mild = +/–, moderate = +, severe = ++

Spreading: Enter No, Uncertain or Yes

* For these items: enter + or –

Making the Diagnosis

History

- Patchy hair loss accompanied with severe itching, pain, and burning is characteristic of LPP, although a few patients with LPP are relatively asymptomatic.

Exam

- The absence of follicular ostia is the clue that this is a cicatricial alopecia and not alopecia areata or androgenetic alopecia. In LPP, hair follicles around the *margins* of the bare areas show perifollicular erythema and perifollicular scale, whereas the center of the bare patches is smooth and devoid of inflammation. This is in contrast to discoid lupus erythematosus (DLE) where the *center* of the bare patches shows inflammation with follicular plugging, erythema, telangiectasia, and varying degrees of hypo- and hyperpigmentation. In alopecia areata, the patches may be distinguished by their peach color and the presence of normal follicular ostia.
- Patients with cicatricial alopecia often have unusually thick hair, or had unusually thick hair before the onset of their cicatricial alopecia.

Scalp Biopsy

- A dense perifollicular lymphocytic infiltrate at the level of the isthmus, decreased sebaceous glands, and scarred fibrous tracts, all support a diagnosis of primary lymphocytic cicatricial alopecia.

The clinical findings together with the histologic picture support a diagnosis of lichen planopilaris.

Discussion

Lichen planopilaris (LPP) is the prototypical lymphocytic cicatricial alopecia. It presents in adults and is more common in women (Fig 1.2). The course is variable. It may evolve slowly with one or more patches of hair loss or diffuse central hair thinning, with slow progression over many years. In other cases, the course is rapid, and within a few months patchy hair loss or diffuse thinning spreads over large areas of the scalp (Fig. 6.2). In all cases, the absence of follicular ostia is the clue that this is a cicatricial alopecia and not alopecia areata or androgenetic alopecia.

LPP is considered a follicular variant of lichen planus (LP) based on clinical and histopathological findings. Cutaneous, nail, and mucous membrane LP may occur before, during, or after the onset of scalp involvement. The occurrence of associated LP varies in reports from 17 to 50% of patients with LPP; at UCSF, about 25% of patients with LPP have had associated cutaneous or mucous membrane LP.

The incidence of any of the cicatricial alopecias is not precisely known. The annual

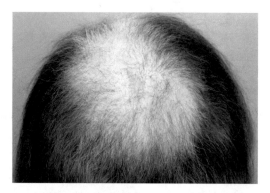

Fig. 6.2 Close up of diffuse LPP with loss of follicular ostia and blotchy erythema

incidence rate of LPP was reported in four tertiary hair research centers in the United States (Figs. 1.1–1.4).

In LPP, symptoms of itching, burning, pain, and tenderness are often severe. The scalp lesions may be single or multiple, focal or diffuse, and can occur anywhere on the scalp. Small bare patches may slowly coalesce with others and enlarge to involve large areas. In a typical active bare area, the center is smooth and devoid of follicular markings. Hair follicles around the *margins* of the bare areas show perifollicular erythema and perifollicular scale (Fig. 6.1). This is in contrast to DLE where the follicular plugging is in the *center* of the active bare patch(es), and in contrast to pseudopelade where there is no perifollicular erythema or perifollicular scale.

A pull test (Fig 2.3) may yield anagen hair in cicatricial alopecia. When present, this is a useful sign of active disease that requires treatment. However, a positive anagen pull test is not always present in active disease, an observation that has not been explained. The loose anchoring of anagen hair in active primary cicatricial alopecia has been considered the result of decreased expression of follicular transglutaminases.

We recommend tracking every patient with cicatricial alopecia with a standardized flow chart at every visit (Table 2.2). The flow chart allows easy documentation of the patient's

---

Table 6.2 Calculation of LPPAI using standardized patient flow chart in Table 6.1

LPPAI (0–10) = (A+B+C+D+E+F)/3 + 2.5(pull test) + 1.5(spreading/2)

A Pruritus *
B Pain *
C Burning *
D Erythema *
E Perifollicular erythema *
F Perifollicular scale *

*Scale for A-F:
−   = 0 => negative
+/− = 1 => questionable or mild
+   = 2 => moderate
++ = 3 => severe

Pull test
no anagen hairs = 0   one or more anagen hairs = 1

Spreading
No = 0
Uncertain = 1
Yes = 2

In the example shown in Table 6.1, the LPPAI for the patient's first visit was calculated as follows:

(3 + 3 + 1 + 3 + 3 + 3)/3 + 2.5(1) + 1.5(2/2) = 9.33

And the LPPAI for the second visit was calculated:

(1 + 1 + 0 +1 + 2 + 2)/3 + 2.5(0) +1.5(0/2) = 2.33

The LPPAI is an equation used to quantify (from 0 to 10) the activity of a patient's LPP at a given time. Eight clinical criteria are included in the LPPAI: pruritus, pain, burning, erythema, perifollicular erythema, perifollicular scale, hair pull test, and spreading. The LPPAI equation was created by weighting the criteria according to subjectivity and observer variability. For example, the hair pull test is the most objective and least variable among clinicians so it received the greatest weight. In addition it was a binary criterion, that is, either positive or negative. The other criteria received a lower weighting because they were either subjective or had greater observer variability.

course and response to treatment over time (otherwise who can remember?) and ensures that nothing has been omitted during patient visits.

Treatment

When the patient is symptomatic, has clinical evidence of disease activity, or has progressive hair loss, systemic medications are recommended. In our view, even a solitary *active* area is an indication for therapy to try to prevent progression (see Chap. 4).

What is the evidence that our current treatments "work" or have any beneficial effect in treating LPP? And what do we mean by "working"? We judge that a drug "works" if it removes symptoms and signs and slows progression. Hair regrowth is not expected and is not a criterion for efficacy in treating cicatricial alopecia. Current empiric treatments do not always slow progression, which may continue insidiously even when symptoms and signs are removed.

Regarding hydroxychloroquine and mycophenolate mofetil, we were uncertain if these drugs were effective in treating LPP because of a lack of a systematic way of monitoring patients while on treatment. A retrospective chart review was conducted on 40 patients with LPP and/or FFA treated with hydroxychloroquine and on 16 patients treated with mycophenolate mofetil. At every visit, numerical values were assigned to symptom severity, to signs including anagen positive pull test, and to progression of hair loss (Table 6.1). This provided the ability to calculate at every visit a single numeric summary of disease activity, the Lichen Planopilaris Activity Index or LPPAI, (scored from 0–10) (Table 6.2). Pre- and post-treatment LPPAI scores were compared using a paired *t* test to determine if there was significant change.

In the review of 40 patients, hydroxychloroquine was significantly effective ($p < 0.001$) in reducing symptoms and signs of active LPP and FFA in 69% and 83% of patients after 6 and 12 months of treatment, respectively.

In the review of 16 patients, mycophenolate mofetil was significantly effective ($p < 0.005$) in reducing symptoms and signs of active LPP in 83% of patients who had failed multiple prior treatments, after 6 months of treatment.

Additional Figures (Figs. 6.3–6.9)

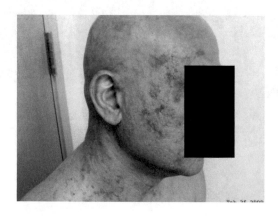

Fig. 6.3 Atrophic LP on the face, follicular LP on the neck and trunk (not shown), and LP on the scalp, as well as cicatricial alopecia on the scalp

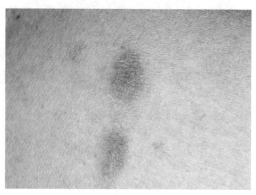

Fig. 6.4 Cutaneous LP (close up) in patient with LPP

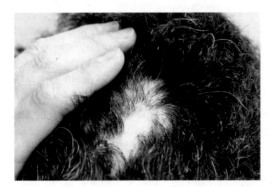

Fig. 6.5 Site of biopsy at hair-bearing margin of active LPP patch

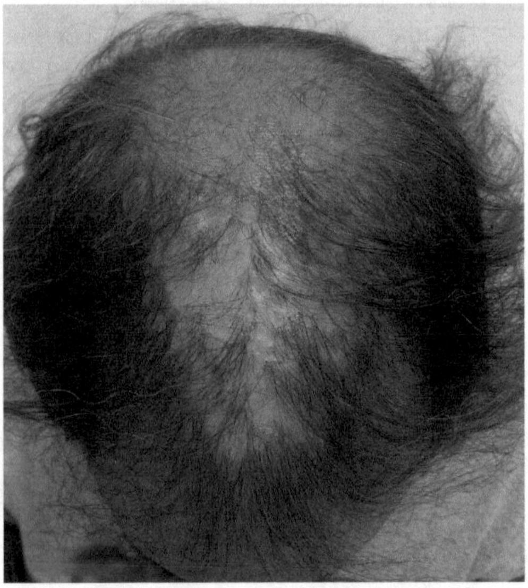

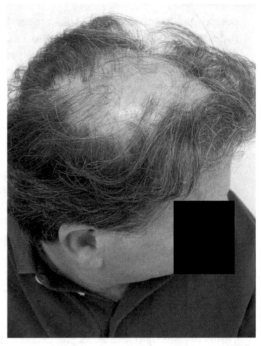

Fig. 6.7 Extensive LPP over large area. Why is this not AGA? Note loss of follicular ostia and sporadic groups of residual terminal hair, absence of miniaturized hairs, blotchy erythema

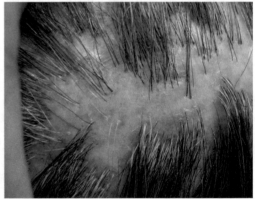

Fig. 6.6 Combination of LPP over frontal scalp and androgenetic alopecia over vertex

Fig. 6.8 Close up of LPP with loss of follicular ostia, blotchy erythema, terminal hair, absence of miniaturized hair, tufted follicles

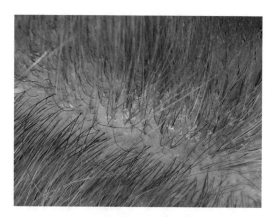

Fig. 6.9 Close-up of LPP with increased spacing between the hair, loss of follicular ostia, perifollicular scaling, and tufted follicles

Takeaway Pearls

> Patchy hair loss accompanied with severe itching, pain, and burning is characteristic of LPP, although a few patients with LPP are relatively asymptomatic.

> In LPP, hair follicles around the *margins* of the bare areas show perifollicular erythema and perifollicular scale, whereas the center of the bare patches is smooth and devoid of inflammation.

> In all cases, the absence of follicular ostia is the clue that this is a cicatricial alopecia and not alopecia areata or androgenetic alopecia.

> Progression of hair loss may continue insidiously even after current treatments have removed all the symptoms and signs.

Suggested Reading

Cevasco NC, Bergfeld WF, Remzi BK, et al. A case-series of 29 patients with lichen planopilaris: the Cleveland Clinic Foundation experience on evaluation, diagnosis and treatment. J Am Acad Dermatol. 2007;57:47–53.

Chiang C, Sah D, Cho BK, et al. Hydroxycholoroquine and lichen planopilaris: efficacy and introduction of Lichen Planopilaris Activity Index scoring system. J Am Acad Dermatol. 2010;62:387–92.

Chieregato C, Zini A, Barba A, et al. Lichen planopilaris: report of 30 cases and review of the literature. Int J Dermatol. 2003;42:342–5.

Cho BK, Sah D, Chwalek J, et al. Efficacy and safety of mycophenolate mofetil for lichen planopilaris. J Am Acad Dermatol. 2010;62:393–7.

Mirmirani P, Karnik P. Lichen planopilaris treated with a peroxisome proliferator-activated receptor gamma agonist. Arch Dermatol. 2009;145:1363–6.

Mirmirani P, Willey A, Price VH. Short course of oral cyclosporine in lichen planopilaris. J Am Acad Dermatol. 2003;49:667–71.

Mirmirani P, Price VH, Karnik P. Decreased expression of follicular transglutaminases: A possible cause for loose anchoring of anagen hair in active primary cicatricial alopecia. J Invest Dermatol. 2008;128 Suppl 1:285.

Ochoa BE, King LE Jr, Price VH. Lichen planopilaris: annual incidence in four hair research centers in the United States. J Am Acad Dermatol. 2008;58:352–3.

Ross EK, Tan E, Shapiro J. Update on primary cicatricial alopecias. J Am Acad Dermatol. 2005;53:1–37.

Tan E, Martinka M, Ball N, et al. Primary cicatricial alopecias: clinicopathology of 112 cases. J Am Acad Dermatol. 2004;50:25–32.

Whiting DA. Cicatricial alopecia: clinico-pathological findings and treatment. Clin Dermatol. 2001;19:211–25.

Graham Little Syndrome

(synonym: Graham Little–Piccardi–Lassueur syndrome)

Clinical Scenario

A 55-year-old woman presents with patchy cicatricial alopecia that has been slowly progressive over 10 years. Five months earlier, she suddenly developed a widespread eruption of papules with spine-like projections on her trunk and limbs. The axillary and pubic hair also disappeared.

Making the Diagnosis

History and Exam

- This rare distinctive syndrome is characterized by the triad of scarring scalp alopecia, widespread keratosis pilaris-like follicular papules on the trunk and limbs, and loss of pubic and axillary hair, which looks nonscarring clinically but histologically shows a scarring process.

Discussion

This syndrome was first described in 1915 by Graham Little in London in a patient referred to him by Lassueur of sp: Lausanne. Piccardi of Italy had described a similar case in the previous year. It is considered a rare variant of LPP.

The three distinctive clinical features include patchy cicatricial alopecia, widespread rapidly developing keratosis pilaris-like follicular papules, and loss of axillary and pubic hair. Clinically, the axillary and pubic hair loss appears nonscarring although histologically there is follicular destruction and scarring. The features may not present simultaneously, and the sequence of events and their relative severity vary widely from case to case. In most reported patients, the earliest change has been patchy cicatricial alopecia. Descriptions of the keratosis pilaris emphasize the conspicuous spiny papules on the trunk and limbs. Most patients have been women between the ages of 30 and 70.

Suggested Reading

Abbas A, Chedraoui A, Ghosn S. Frontal fibrosing alopecia presenting with components of Piccardi–Lassueur–Graham Little syndrome. J Am Acad Dermatol. 2007; 57:515–8.

Bianchi l, Paro Vidolin A, Piemonte P, et al. Graham–Little–Piccardi–Lassueur syndrome: effective treatment with cyclosporin A. Clin Exp Dermatol. 2001; 26:518–20.

Dawber RPR, Fenton DA. Cicatricial alopecia. In: Dawber R, editor. Diseases of the hair and scalp. 3rd ed. Oxford: Blackwell; 1997:370–96.

Frontal Fibrosing Alopecia

Clinical Scenario

A 64-year-old Caucasian patient consults her dermatologist because her hairline is receding. Five years earlier, she noticed thinning of her right eyebrow and 2 years later noticed gradual recession of her frontal hairline. She has mild itching. A scalp exam shows very thick curly hair that reaches her shoulders. The frontal hairline has receded 2 cm, and there is diminishment of

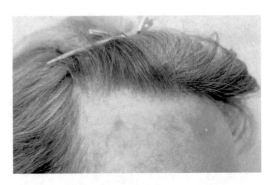

Fig. 6.10 Frontal fibrosing alopecia in a 64-year-old woman showing hairline recession demarcated by the photodamage of the lower forehead

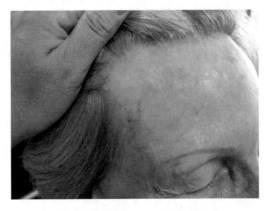

Fig. 6.11 Frontal fibrosing alopecia with loss of eyebrows (only right brow shown). With permission: Fu JM, Price VH. Cicatricial alopecia. J Dermatol Nurses' Assoc. 2010;2:1–5

follicular markings in the receded area (Fig. 6.10). The remaining terminal hairs in the affected area show perifollicular erythema. The hairline recession is demarcated by the photodamage on the lower forehead below the original hairline. Both eyebrows have patchy thinning (Fig. 6.11). The dermatologist advised a scalp biopsy.

Making the Diagnosis

History

• Recession of the frontal/temporal hairline associated with loss of the eyebrows are characteristic features of frontal fibrosing cicatricial alopecia.

Exam

- The 2 cm frontal hairline recession with diminishment of follicular markings and perifollicular erythema suggest FFA rather than alopecia areata. Her very thick hair is a common finding in patients with primary cicatricial alopecia.

Scalp Biopsy

- A dense lymphocytic infiltrate surrounding the isthmus is present.

The clinical and histologic findings together support a diagnosis of FFA.

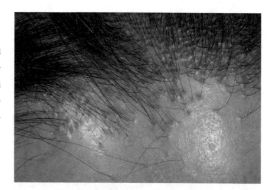

Fig. 6.12 Frontal fibrosing alopecia with prominent perifollicular erythema

Discussion

FFA is characterized by a distinctive clinical pattern of progressive recession of the frontal/temporal hairline often associated with progressive loss of eyebrows. Although the latter might suggest alopecia areata, the presence of perifollicular erythema (Fig. 6.12) and decreased follicular markings support FFA. FFA was first described by Kossard in 1994 in postmenopausal women, and it was thought to be a mild variant of LPP. Since then cases have been reported in premenopausal women (Fig. 6.13), as well as a few cases in men. Moreover, we now know that the distinct clinical presentations of the lymphocytic cicatricial alopecias look similar histologically, and in our opinion FFA is a separate entity and not a variant of LPP. Recently, the number of new cases of FFA appears to be increasing, and in our centers, the number of new cases is now greater than the new cases of all the other lymphocytic cicatricial alopecias.

Skin along the hairline is pale and contrasts with the photo-damaged skin of the lower forehead, with the line of demarcation indicating the location of the original hairline (Fig. 6.10). In some patients, the pale skin of the receded hairline appears atrophic. The band-like frontal recession may progress laterally to above and behind the ears and less often to the occipital hairline.

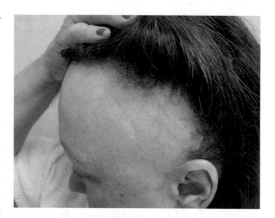

Fig. 6.13 Frontal fibrosing alopecia in a younger woman with 3 cm frontal-temporal hairline recession and diminished eyebrows (only left brow shown)

The recession varies from 1 to 6 cm. It may be slow in spreading, sometimes is self-limited, or may be rapidly progressive. Rarely, the frontal recession can progress posteriorly as far back as the center of the scalp as well as behind the ears to the occipital hairline (Fig. 6.14). Perifollicular erythema at the receding hairline is a helpful sign and indicates active follicular inflammation. Perifollicular scale is usually slight or absent in FFA. Prominence of veins on the forehead may be seen in patients with FFA, including those who have never received intralesional corticosteroids. Many patients have itching, but generally FFA is less symptomatic than LPP.

Loss of eyebrows may be complete or partial and is supportive of the diagnosis of FFA. It appears at the same time as the hairline recession in most cases; however, it may precede the

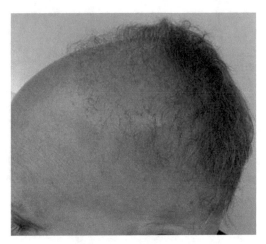

Fig. 6.14 Extensive frontal recession extending to the vertex with spreading above and behind the ears to the occipital hairline

Table 6.3 Frontal fibrosing alopecia patient demographics and clinical findings

Category	No. (%)	Median (range)
Total no. of patients	36 (100)	
Age of onset (years)		59 (30–79)
Women	35 (97.2)	
Age of onset (years)		59 (30–79)
Men	1 (2.8)	
Age of onset (years)		47
Ethnicity		
Caucasian	33 (91.7)	
African-American	2(5.5)	
Asian (Oriental)	1 (2.8)	
Menopausal status of women		
Premenopausal	6 (17.1)	
Postmenopausal	29 (82.8)	
Concurrent or prior lichen planus		
Oral	1 (2.8)	
Vulval	1 (2.8)	
Cutaneous	1 (2.8)	
Symptoms at onset		
Pruritus	24 (66.7)	
Pain	6 (16.7)	
Burning	3 (8.3)	
Anagen pull test		
Positive	17 (47.2)	
Additional site(s) of alopecia		
Eyebrows	27 (75)	
Eyelashes	3 (8.3)	
Upper limbs	7 (19.4)	
Lower limbs	6 (16.7)	
Axilla	1 (2.8)	
Pubic area	0 (0)	

With permission: Samrao A, Chew A, Price VH. Frontal fibrosing alopecia: a clinical review of 36 patients. Br J Dermatol. 2010; 163:1296–300

hairline recession by years, or appear after the onset. Patients may also report loss of limb hair, and loss of eyelashes. Histologic findings in FFA are indistinguishable from those of LPP and the other lymphocytic cicatricial alopecias (See Chap. 3).

Lichen planopilaris may develop in some patients with FFA. Cutaneous or mucous membrane lichen planus may also occur but is less common in patients with FFA than in patients with LPP.

At present, there is no explanation for the curious association of frontal hairline recession and associated eyebrow loss and occasional limb and eyelash loss. Histology of affected eyebrows and limbs has shown a scarring process rather than features of alopecia areata.

The increased incidence of this acquired, non-hereditary, distinctive cicatricial alopecia described for the first time in 1994 has been noted in North America, Europe, and Australia. We suspect that an environmental factor may be involved in FFA, and if so, it appears to have an affinity for the pilosebaceous follicle.

A review of the clinical features of 36 patients with FFA (35 females and 1 male) is shown in Table 6.3.

Treatment

See Chap. 4 for medical management of FFA.

For Treatment of Eyebrow Loss in FFA

We offer intralesional corticosteroids with triamcinolone acetonide, 10 mg/cc, and inject a maximum total of 0.25 cc to the two brows, with five or six tiny injections with a 30-gauge needle to each brow. This is repeated at 6-week to 3-month intervals. How effective are these brow injections? In a review of ten patients with FFA and eyebrow loss who were treated with intralesional triamcinolone acetonide, nine responded with some measure of hair growth (see Fig 6.15).

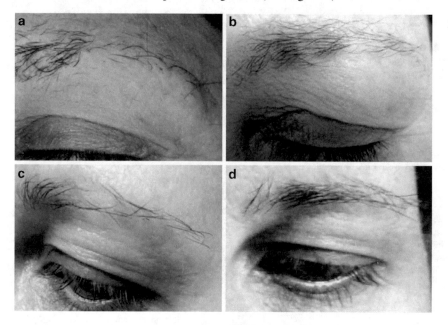

Fig. 6.15 Eyebrow regrowth in two patients with frontal fibrosing alopecia treated with intralesional injections of triamcinolone acetonide (10 mg/cc). (a) and (b) 45-year-old woman following nine injections over 27 months. (c) and (d) 41-year-old woman following eight injections over 11 months. With permission: Donovan JC, Samrao A, Ruben BS, et al. Eyebrow regrowth in frontal fibrosing alopecia patients treated with intralesional triamcinolone acetonadie. Br J Dermatol. 2010; 163:1142–4

Additional Figures (Figs. 6.16–6.19)

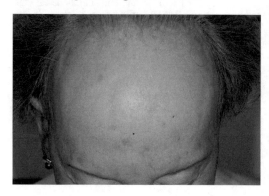

Fig. 6.16 Extensive hairline recession with bilateral eyebrow loss

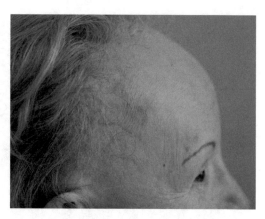

Fig. 6.17 Extensive hairline recession with loss of right eyebrow. Note prominence of temporal veins that may be seen in patients with FFA, including those who have never received intralesional corticosteroid. In some patients, the pale skin of the receded hairline may appear atrophic along with loss of follicular markings

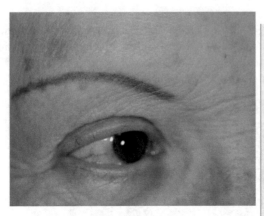

Fig. 6.18 Absent eyebrow and diminished eyelashes in a patient with frontal fibrosing alopecia

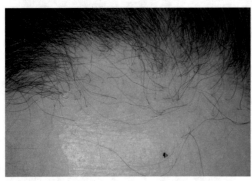

Fig. 6.19 Frontal fibrosing alopecia with increased curliness of remaining hairs due to dermal fibrosis. Note absent follicular ostia

> Loss of eyebrows may be reversible with intralesional triamcinolone acetonide injections in patients who still have some remaining brows.
> An increased incidence of this acquired, nonhereditary, distinctive cicatricial alopecia described for the first time in 1994 has been noted in North America, Europe, and Australia.
> If an environmental factor is involved in FFA, it appears to have an affinity for hair follicles.

Suggested Reading

Donovan JC, Samrao A, Ruben BS, et al. Eyebrow regrowth in frontal fibrosing alopecia patients treated with triamcinolone acetonide injection. Br J Dermatol. 2010;163:1142–44.

Kossard S. Postmenopausal frontal fibrosing alopecia. Scarring alopecia in a pattern distribution. Arch Dermatol. 1994;130:770–4.

Kossard S. Postmenopausal frontal fibrosing alopecia: a frontal variant of lichen planopilaris. J Am Acad Dermatol. 1997;36:59–66.

Miteva M, Camacho I, Romanelli P, et al. Acute hair loss on the limbs in Frontal Fibrosing Alopecia: A clinicopathological study of two cases. Br J Dermatol. 2010; 163:426–8.

Moreno-Ramirez D, Camacho Martinez F. Frontal fibrosing alopecia: A survey of 16 patients. J Eur Acad Dermatol Venereol. 2005;19:700–5.

Naz E, Vidaurrazaga C, Hernandez-Cano N, et al. Postmenopausal frontal fibrosing alopecia. Clin Exp Dermatol. 2003;28:25–7.

Ross EK, Tan E, Shapiro J. Update on primary cicatricial alopecias. J Am Acad Dermatol. 2005;53:1–37.

Samrao A, Chew A, Price VH. Frontal fibrosing alopecia: A clinical review of 36 patients. Br J Dermatol. 2010;163:1296–300.

Whiting DA. Cicatricial alopecia: clinico-pathological findings and treatment. Clin Dermatol. 2001; 19:211–25.

Takeaway Pearls

> *Clinical manifestations.* Band-like pattern of recession along frontal, temporal, and (less commonly) occipital hairline associated with loss of the eyebrows.
> Loss of eyebrows may precede the hairline recession by years, or occur at the same time, or appear after the onset.
> Skin along the receding frontal hairline is pale and contrasts with the photo-damaged skin of the lower forehead; the line of demarcation indicates the location of the original hairline.
> Perifollicular erythema at the receding hairline is a helpful sign; perifollicular scale is usually slight or absent in FFA.

Pseudopelade (Brocq)

Clinical Scenario

A 56-year-old Caucasian woman presents for a second opinion. Her hairdresser noted small patches of hair loss approximately 6 months ago.

The patient consulted a dermatologist and was told she had alopecia areata. However, after three treatments with intralesional triamcinolone acetonide injections there has been no hair regrowth, and new patches of hair loss have appeared. The patient has no symptoms. On exam, there are small, 1–2 cm patches of hair loss along the central part of the scalp. The patches are white, smooth, and devoid of follicular markings. There is no inflammation of the scalp. The patient's eyebrows, eyelashes, and fingernails appear normal. A scalp biopsy is taken.

Making the Diagnosis

History

- Patients with pseudopelade (Brocq) (PPB) present with patchy hair loss that is generally asymptomatic.

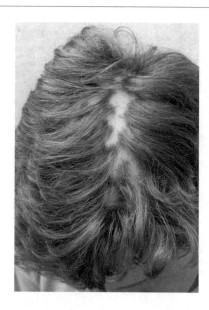

Fig. 6.20 Pseudopelade (Brocq) resembling alopecia areata, but note that the patches are irregular in shape, not round or oval, follicular ostia are absent, and the scalp is white in this light-skinned patient rather than peach colored. There is no erythema or scaling

Exam

- Patches of hair loss in PPB are often mistaken for alopecia areata.
- In contrast to alopecia areata, the patches of hair loss in PPB are devoid of follicular markings, have an irregular shape, are not round or oval, and in light-skinned persons the scalp is white rather than peach-colored as in alopecia areata (Figs. 6.20–6.23).
- In light-skinned persons, the pattern of hair loss has been described as resembling "footprints in the snow."

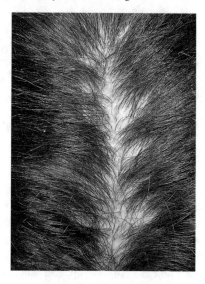

Fig. 6.21 Pseudopelade (Brocq) resembling alopecia areata, but note irregular shape of the patchy loss, absent follicular ostia, and the white appearance of the affected scalp. Absent clinical inflammation

Biopsy

- Moderate perifollicular lymphocytic infiltrate at the level of the follicular infundibulum; sebaceous glands are reduced; reduced numbers of follicles and replacement with fibrous tracts.

The clinical presentation and histologic findings support a diagnosis of pseudopelade (Brocq).

Discussion

Pseudopelade as described by Brocq (PPB) over a 100 years ago is a rare primary lymphocyte-mediated cicatricial alopecia characterized by

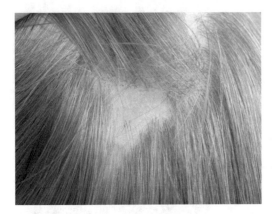

Fig. 6.22 Pseudopelade (Brocq) resembling alopecia areata, but note irregular shape, not round, absent follicular ostia, and white appearance of the scalp. No erythema or scaling

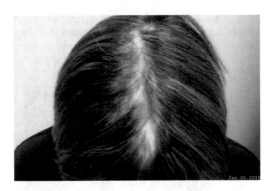

Fig. 6.23 Pseudopelade (Brocq) resembling alopecia areata. Note irregular shape of patchy loss and white appearance of the scalp

small patchy areas of hair loss. "Pelade" is the French term for alopecia areata, and the name "pseudopelade" emphasizes the resemblance to alopecia areata (Figs. 6.20–6.22). In the literature, the debate continues whether PPB is a distinct clinical entity or an end stage of many cicatricial alopecias. This debate stems mainly from the inability of authors to distinguish PPB from LPP histologically. These authors have not accepted that the histology of the primary cicatricial alopecias cannot distinguish the clinical subtypes: histopathology can only distinguish two groups: the predominantly lymphocytic group and the predominantly neutrophilic group. An additional factor causing the debate is that in PPB there are few or no clinical signs of

inflammation, hence the resemblance to alopecia areata. However, PPB is a distinct acute stage disease and is histologically indistinguishable from LPP and the other lymphocyte-mediated cicatricial alopecias. Recent microarray analysis compared the gene expression profiles of LPP and PPB and clearly indicated that PPB is a distinct active disease and not a late- or end-stage phase of LPP.

We urge readers to abandon using the term "pseudopelade" to describe end-stage nonspecific cicatricial alopecia. Instead, the preferred terminology is pseudopelade (Brocq) (PPB) to describe the primary lymphocytic cicatricial alopecia, as detailed in this chapter, and the term "end-stage nonspecific cicatricial alopecia" to describe end stage of any primary cicatricial alopecia when the clinical features are no longer distinguishable and histology shows sparse hair follicles, many scarred fibrous tracts, and absent sebaceous glands (see "End-stage nonspecific cicatricial alopecia" in Chap. 9).

PPB has its onset in adulthood and does not seem to have any racial predilection. The typical clinical presentation is of multiple discrete, small, smooth bare patches with no inflammation; the irregular shapes extend in an asymmetric, irregular manner. In light-skinned persons, the patches are white- or ivory-colored and have been described as "footprints in the snow." The small patches of alopecia may coalesce to form larger patches, and there may be a combination of small and large patches on the scalp. The course is slowly progressive. Residual solitary hairs in the bare patch may be kinky or curly, a feature thought to be due to follicular torsion as a result of dermal fibrosis (Fig. 6.24). Tufted follicles may be seen, although this is not usually a pronounced feature in PPB.

In contrast to PPB, in central centrifugal cicatricial alopecia (CCCA) alopecia, the hair loss starts as a central patch at the vertex or upper occipital scalp and spreads in a symmetrical and centrifugal manner; however, both PPB and CCCA may be asymptomatic and both have diminished follicular ostia. In lichen planopilaris, the patches of hair loss show perifollicular scaling and perifollicular erythema at the margins and loss of follicular ostia; LPP is usually very symptomatic. In alopecia

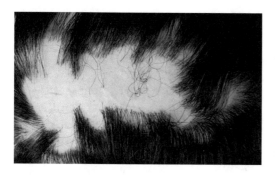

Fig. 6.24 Pseudopelade (Brocq) with ivory white scalp, absent follicular ostia, and kinking of the hair attributed to dermal fibrosis that causes torsion of the follicles. Note absence of erythema or scaling

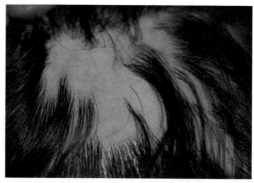

Fig. 6.26 Pseudopelade (Brocq) with confluent bare patches, absent follicular ostia, tufted follicles, mild blotchy pinkness

areata, the follicular markings are intact, and the patches are often peach-colored (see Table 9.1).

The course of PPB is one of progressive hair loss which may be slow or rapid, with periods of quiescence and intermittent flares. Management of PPB is the same as described in Chap. 4 for the lymphocytic cicatricial alopecias. However, assessing clinical activity and treatment response in PPB is more challenging because of the absence of clinical signs and symptoms. For this reason, measurements of areas of hair loss when practical, photographs, and repeated biopsies are used to choose treatment and to gauge response (see "Discussion" in Chap. 9) .

Additional Figures (Figs. 6.25 and 6.26)

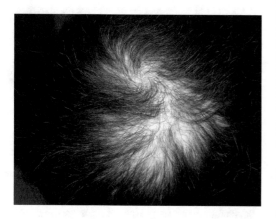

Fig. 6.25 Pseudopelade (Brocq) with patchy hair loss, loss of follicular ostia, and mild blotchy pinkness

Takeaway PPB Pearls

> PPB clinically resembles alopecia areata (AA) because of asymptomatic patchy or scaling.

> To differentiate PPB and AA: In PPB, follicular ostia are diminished and in light-skinned individuals the patches of hair loss are white resembling "footprints in the snow." In AA, follicular ostia are normal and the patches of hair loss are are often peach-colored.

> Residual solitary hairs in a bare patch may be kinky or curly, a feature thought to be due to follicular torsion as a result of dermal fibrosis.

> Recommendation that the term "pseudopelade" not be used to describe late, end-stage nonspecific cicatricial alopecia.

> Preferred terminology is pseudopelade (Brocq) (PPB) to describe the primary lymphocytic cicatricial alopecia, as detailed in this chapter, and the term "end-stage nonspecific cicatricial alopecia" to describe late or end stage of any primary cicatricial alopecia.

Suggested Reading

Annessi G, Lombardo G. Gobello T, et al. A clinico-pathologic study of scarring alopecia due to lichen planus: comparison with scarring alopecia in discoid lupus erythematosus and pseudopelade. Am J Dermatopathol. 1999;21:324–31.

Dawber RPR, Fenton DA. Cicatricial alopecia. In: Dawber R, editor. Diseases of the hair and scalp. 3rd ed. Oxford: Blackwell; 1997:370–96.

Mirmirani P, Willey A, Headington JT, et al. Primary cicatricial alopecia: histological findings do not distinguish clinical variants. J Am Acad Dermatol. 2005;52:637–43.

Nayer M, Schomberg K, Dawber RP, et al. A clinico-pathological study of scarring alopecia. Br J Dermatol. 1993;128:533–6.

Ross EK, Tan E, Shapiro J. Update on primary cicatricial alopecias. J Am Acad Dermatol. 2005; 53:1–37.

Tan E, Martinka M, Ball N, et al. Primary cicatricial alopecias: clinicopathology of 112 cases. J Am Acad Dermatol. 2004;50:25–32.

Whiting DA. Cicatricial alopecia: clinico-pathological findings and treatment. Clin Dermatol. 2001;19:211–25.

Yu M, Bell RH, Ross EK, et al. Lichen planopilaris and pseudopelade of Brocq involve distinct disease associated gene expression patterns by microarray. J Dermatol Sci. 2010;57:27–36.

Central Centrifugal Cicatricial Alopecia

Clinical Scenario

A 47-year-old African American woman presents with severe scalp itching and a 7-year history of hair breaking and hair thinning along the scalp margins. She also has noted hair thinning over her vertex for 3–4 years. For over 10 years, she has had the nightly practice of wrapping her hair tightly on top of her head before going to bed. She had frequent perms in the past but not in the past year. There is no other relevant medical history, and the patient is otherwise healthy.

On examination, she has a very short haircut and obvious thinning along the margins of her scalp. Over the vertex, there is increased spacing between the hairs and diminished follicular markings. Moderate scaling is present throughout the scalp. A pull test cannot be done because the hair is too fragile and breaks. A tug test breaks off short bits of hair, which are saved in a paper envelope for later mounting. A 4-mm scalp punch biopsy is taken from the thinning scalp vertex, and laboratory tests are ordered: CBC, TSH, ferritin, and Vitamin D 25OH.

Making the Diagnosis

History

- The presentation suggests four separate problems: hair breakage, traction alopecia, possible early CCCA, and seborrheic dermatitis.

Exam

- The short broken bits of hair are mounted in Permount®, and with low-power light microscopy they show trichorrhexis nodosa fractures and longitudinal splitting (Fig. 6.27), correlating with the marked hair fragility and breakage demonstrated clinically with a tug test.
- Her thinning hair along the frontal/temporal hair margins represents traction alopecia and is related to her 10-year nightly practice of tightly wrapping her hair on top of her head.
- Her severe scalp itching is probably caused by the seborrheic dermatitis.
- Laboratory tests show ferritin 10 and vitamin D 25OH 14, and normal CBC and TSH.

Biopsy

- Scalp biopsy from the vertex shows a lymphocyte-mediated primary scarring alopecia with a moderate peri-infundibular lymphocytic infiltrate and fibrosis; sebaceous glands are diminished.

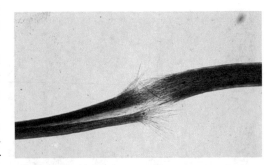

Fig. 6.27 Hair mount of broken hair from a tug test showing trichorrhexis nodosa and longitudinal spitting (Mounted in Permount ®). With permission: Price VH. Structural anomalies of the hair shaft. In: Orfanos CE and Happle R, editors. Hair and hair diseases. New York: Springer; 1990. p. 363–422

The clinical and histologic findings support a diagnosis of CCCA. In addition, this patient has hair fragility and hair breakage confirmed by the positive tug test and hair mount showing trichorrhexis nodosa. She has traction alopecia in keeping with her history and hair thinning along the hair margins. The generalized scalp scaling is due to seborrheic dermatitis. She has low ferritin and low vitamin D 25OH and will be given appropriate supplements.

Discussion

CCCA occurs typically in women of African ancestry, usually between the ages of 25 and 65 years. The chief complaint is usually, "I am losing my hair," but women of color may have more than one hair problem, and for this reason it is helpful to begin, somewhat unconventionally, with a clinical exam of the hair and scalp before taking the history. Hair breakage or traction alopecia may also be present in a patient with CCCA, and if present, this needs to be addressed separately. This initial exam helps to guide the subsequent history taking to the most relevant questions.

The cause of CCCA is unknown. Genetic predisposition is likely a factor. Women with CCCA may have female relatives with a similar problem, which makes CCCA the only cicatricial alopecia in which family members (usually female relatives) may have a similar problem. Men have also been reported with CCCA, although the frequency is much lower than in women (Fig 1.2). Currently, the debated and unresolved question is what role the unique grooming and hair styling practices of women with African ancestry play in causing CCCA. Chemical relaxers, heat, and traction are suspected agents. It has been postulated that follicular stem cells may be repeatedly injured by chemical, thermal, and physical trauma over many years. However, many women with African ancestry who have used the same styling practices for many years do not have CCCA, and some women with CCCA have never used chemical relaxers. An ongoing survey indicates that only a small percentage of women who have used chemical relaxers have CCCA, which suggests that hair care practices alone are not the cause of CCCA. A combination of genetic and environmental factors may predispose some women to CCCA. Indeed, it is noteworthy that the histology of CCCA is indistinguishable from the histology of the other lymphocyte-mediated cicatricial alopecias, suggesting that CCCA is a common pathway of various causes in genetically predisposed women.

Questions directed at CCCA include: when did you or your hairdresser first notice any hair problem? Did the hair loss begin centrally and then spread symmetrically in all directions? Do any other women in the family have a similar problem? Have you experienced itching, pain, tenderness, burning, scaling? Is the hair loss still spreading compared to 1 year ago, or has it stabilized?

Questions directed at hair breakage: If hair breakage is present, a history of hair care practices is essential. Ask if she uses or has used relaxers or perms, how often? Does she use heat in the form of hot combs, hot rollers, ceramic flat irons? Does she brush her hair "to stimulate hair that will not grow long"? What kind of brush does she use? Natural bristle brushes are more damaging to hair than plastic bristles with rounded tips (not knobs). Is the scalp itchy or scaly and does this cause much scratching and rubbing?

Questions directed at traction alopecia: If traction alopecia also appears to be present, ask if she is aware of hair thinning above the ears and behind the frontal hairline. For how many years has this been present? Does she style her hair pulled back? Did she wear it pulled back in the past? Does she sleep with rollers? Has she worn braids or ponytails for any extended period in childhood or later?

With CCCA, associated symptoms are usually mild, if any, but episodic itching or tenderness may occur. Patients first note thinning over a small area of the central scalp (Fig. 6.28). This gradually enlarges centrifugally in a symmetrical manner and may affect a large area on the top with extension to the sides of the scalp (Fig. 6.29). The

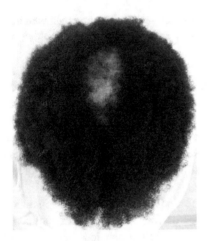

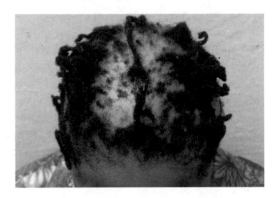

Fig. 6.30 CCCA in a young girl with dramatic increased curliness attributed to torsional forces caused by extensive dermal fibrosis

Fig. 6.28 Central centrifugal alopecia starts on the central scalp with little inflammation

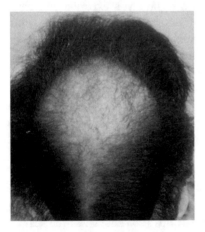

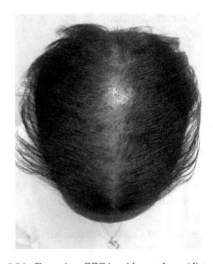

Fig. 6.29 CCCA spreads centrifugally in a symmetric manner with little inflammation and loss of follicular ostia

Fig. 6.31 Extensive CCCA with patulous (distended) follicles. Biopsy is needed to rule out co-existing female pattern thinning

scalp is usually not inflamed. Sparse terminal hairs remain in the affected areas; some may show increased curliness, a result of torsional forces caused by the extensive dermal fibrosis (Fig. 6.30). The affected scalp shows loss of follicular ostia, with residual ostia appearing patulous (distended) and often dusky (Fig. 6.31).

Check for hair breakage: Suspect breakage if there are hairs of varying lengths with blunt distal ends; ask the patient if the hair has been purposely cut in layers, which would give a similar appearance. Hair that is breaking is fragile. To demonstrate fragility, do a "tug test": grasp a cluster of hairs with the thumb and index finger

of one hand and tug at their distal ends with the thumb and index finger of the other hand (Fig 2.7). Fragile hair breaks into small bits, which show characteristic fractures in a hair mount (Fig. 6.27).

Check for traction alopecia: is there thinning/receding of the temporal or frontal hairline? The main differential diagnosis is alopecia areata. Traction alopecia can be differentiated from alopecia areata by the "fringe sign," the presence of terminal hairs outlining the original hairline, a finding not usually seen in alopecia areata; sparse terminal hairs remain in the receded area (Fig. 6.32).

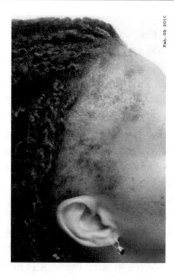

Fig. 6.32 Traction alopecia in a patient with CCCA (wearing extensions). Note the "fringe sign": terminal hairs that outline the original hairline. Sparse terminal hairs remain in the receded area

Treatment

For CCCA

CCCA needs to be explained to the patient as a condition that affects primarily women of African ancestry and causes hair loss that is permanent, but has no other effect on general health. The cause is unknown. It is not the patient's fault nor the hairdresser's fault. Explain that the role of hair care products in CCCA is being studied and no conclusion has been reached yet. At present, it appears that a combination of genetic and environmental factors may predispose some women to CCCA. The patient will appreciate the discussion and your awareness of the impact that her hair loss has on her daily life.

If the patient reports ongoing spreading of the hair loss and the scalp biopsy shows activity, with a moderate to dense perifollicular lymphocytic infiltrate, we use systemic therapy as well as topical therapy (see Chap. 4). The margins of the affected areas, including the surrounding normal-looking scalp, should be treated with topical therapy to try to control further extension of the inflammation and hair loss. If the patient has not noted continued spreading of the hair

loss and the scalp biopsy shows primarily dermal fibrosis and little or no inflammatory infiltrate, then medical therapy will contribute little. Discuss cosmetic options available to her including hair extensions and creative hair styling (Figs. 6.33–6.36). She may continue to color her hair, and she will be grateful for your concern and input about these issues.

For hair breakage: Patients who state that their hair has "has stopped growing" may not be aware the hair is breaking. It helps explain that the hair is breaking because it has become very fragile and resembles threads of spun glass. Hair fragility and breakage usually result from the cumulative effect

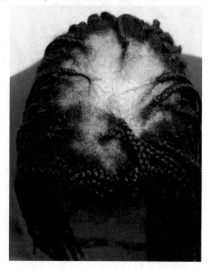

Fig. 6.33 Cosmetic solution for extensive CCCA: hair extensions to mask the hair loss

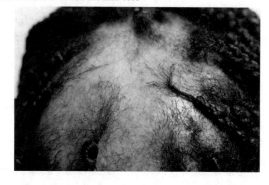

Fig. 6.34 Note the proper attachment of extensions that do not pull the hair as it exits the scalp (absence of "tenting" of the scalp). With permission: Fu JM and Price VH. Cicatricial Alopecia. Journal Dermatol Nurs Assoc. 2010;2:1–5

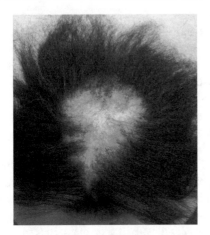

Fig. 6.35 For a cosmetic solution for extensive CCCA, see Fig 6.36

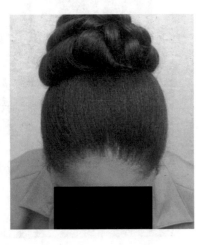

Fig. 6.36 Cosmetic solution for patient in Fig 6.35: creative hair styling

of hair care practices. In some patients, hair is fragile from an early age and in others hair breakage occurs for the first time much later in life. The solution is not simple or easy for the patient. The use of chemical perms and relaxers, excessive heat, brushing "to stimulate hair growth," bristle brushes, vigorous massages should be avoided. A compromise may be to decrease the use of chemical relaxers to every 10–12 weeks. The use of heat, including hot combs, hot rollers, ceramic flat irons, must be minimized. A silicone-containing conditioner may soften the hair and allow it to bend without breaking. Hair pieces or wigs allow the hair to rest because all hair care practices can stop. Many patients need reassurance that a wig

will not cause more damage, and will not affect the blood supply to the hair. An alternative way to rest the hair is to use extensions providing they do not pull the hair tightly as it exits the scalp (Fig. 6.34). Visible bare areas can be camouflaged with powders, creams, mascara, and sprays. It often takes 2–4 years before fragile hair starts to grow normally, even after chemical, heat, and mechanical factors have been appropriately decreased or discontinued.

For traction alopecia, excessive traction or pull on the hair must be avoided. Ponytails, braids, and corn rows are permitted as long as they are loose and do not pull on the hair. You should check to see if the braids or corn rows pull the skin up as it exits the scalp (so-called "tenting"); this must be avoided. Recent onset traction alopecia is reversible as long as the causative hair care practices are avoided. Long-standing traction alopecia may be permanent.

Finally, explain that stopping the above hair styling and grooming practices addresses the hair breakage and traction alopecia and has no effect on the CCCA.

For patients with end-stage CCCA that has been stable for 2 or more years, surgical options may be considered.

Additional Figures (Figs. 6.37 and 6.38)

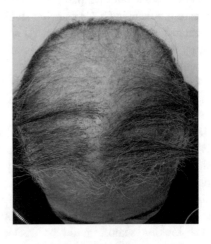

Fig. 6.37 Extensive CCCA showing marked irregular spacing between the hairs, patulous (distended) follicles, and mild blotchy erythema. Biopsy is needed to rule out co-existing female pattern hair loss

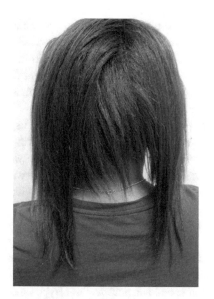

Fig. 6.38   Hair breakage from the use of ceramic flat irons

Takeaway Pearls

> Occurs typically in women of African ancestry and starts as a small area of thinning at vertex or upper occipital scalp.

> Hair loss gradually extends centrifugally in a symmetrical manner.

> Often asymptomatic but itching can vary from mild to severe.

> Little or no signs of inflammation, unless seborrheic dermatitis also present.

> If itching suddenly becomes a predominant symptom, inquire about exposure to children who have tinea capitis.

> Hair breakage and/or traction alopecia may occur in a patient with CCCA, and if present need to be addressed separately.

> Distinguish traction alopecia from alopecia areata by the "fringe sign," the presence of terminal hairs outlining the original hairline.

Suggested Reading

Callender VD. African American scalp disorders and treatment considerations. Skin Aging. 2002;10(S):12–4.

Callender VD, McMichael AJ, Cohen GF. Medical and surgical therapies for alopecias in black women. Dermatol Ther. 2004;17:164–76.

Fu JM, Price VH. Approach to hair loss in women of color. Semin Cutan Med Surg. 2009;28:109–14.

Gathers RC, Lim HW. Central centrifugal cicatricial alopecia: past, present, and future. J Am Acad Dermatol. 2009;60:660–8.

Gathers RC, Jankowski M, Eide M, et al. Hair grooming practices and central centrifugal cicatricial alopecia. J Am Acad Dermatol. 2009;60:574–8.

Khumalo NP. Grooming and central centrifugal cicatricial alopecia. J Am Acad Dermatol. 2010;62:507–8.

Khumalo NP, Jessop S, Gumedze F, et al. Hairdressing is associated with scalp disease in African schoolchildren. Br J Dermatol. 2007;157:106–10.

Khumalo NP, Jessop S, Gumedze F, et al. Hairdressing and the prevalence of scalp disease in African adults. Br J Dermatol. 2007;157(5):981–8.

Khumalo NP, Pillay K, Ngwanya RM. Acute 'relaxer'-associated scarring alopecia: a report of five cases. Br J Dermatol. 2007;156:1394–7.

McMichael AJ. Ethnic hair updates: past and present. J Am Acad Dermatol. 2003;48:S127–33.

Olsen EA, Callender V, McMichael A, et al. Central hair loss in African American women: incidence and potential risk factors. J Am Acad Dermatol. 2011;64:245–52.

Ross EK, Tan E, Shapiro J. Update on primary cicatricial alopecias. J Am Acad Dermatol. 2005;53:1–37.

Chronic Cutaneous Lupus Erythematosus

Clinical Scenario

A 61-year-old African American woman presents with a several year history of patchy scalp hair thinning as well as itching, redness, and scaling predominantly over the posterior scalp. She also reports itching and redness in the ears. On exam, she has diffuse fine scaling with multiple 1–3 cm erythematous scaly patches with surrounding hypo- and hyperpigmentation. Pull test is negative. On the occipital scalp, there are two 1–2 cm bare areas with a smooth surface and absent follicular ostia. In the inner helices of both ears, there is mottled hypo- and hyperpigmentation and follicular plugging. DLE is suspected with both acute and chronic phases noted. A work-up for systemic lupus has been negative in the past. A scalp biopsy is taken.

Making the Diagnosis

History

- Patchy hair loss in an African American woman associated with redness and itching on the scalp as well as in the ears suggests that discoid lupus must be considered.

Exam

- Hypo- and hyperpigmentation around scaly erythematous scalp patches, and follicular plugging and hypo- and hyperpigmentation in the inner helices of the ears suggest DLE.

Scalp biopsy

- A superficial and deep perivascular and peri-adnexal lymphoplasmacytic infiltrate (most prominent around eccrine coils) is noted. Prominent vacuolar change is noted at the dermal–epidermal junction with marked thickening of the epidermal basement membrane. There is near total lack of pilosebaceous units. These findings support a scarring alopecia due to lupus erythematosus.

The clinical and histologic findings support a diagnosis of DLE.

Discussion

CCLE is not a primary cicatricial alopecia but rather a cutaneous manifestation of the autoimmune spectrum of lupus erythematosus (Chap. 5). Within CCLE are three major forms: the most common is DLE, and the less common forms are lupus panniculitis/profundus and lupus tumidus. In none of these forms is the hair follicle the *target* of a folliculocentric inflammatory attack. In DLE, the inflammation is not only perifollicular but also vacuolar at the dermal–epidermal junction, perivascular, and

periadnexal (especially around eccrine coils). If treated early, it is potentially reversible. The clinical presentation of DLE may simulate LPP, and because this presents an important differential diagnosis, we include it to emphasize the differentiating features.

DLE is more common in women, especially women of African ancestry. It may occur at any age but onset is frequent in persons between age 20 and 40 years. Few patients (5–10%) with DLE progress to SLE, although in patients with classic SLE, DLE occurs in about 20% of patients.

DLE most commonly affects the scalp, face, and ears. It starts as a well-demarcated scaly purplish macule or papule and enlarges into a discoid (coin-shaped) alopecic patch with follicular plugging, erythema, and adherent scaling. Hypo- and hyper-pigmentation, telangiectasia, and follicular plugging are characteristics of DLE and are not typically found in the primary cicatricial alopecias; these features are seen in the *center* of the affected patches and are helpful in making the diagnosis of DLE (Figs. 6.39–6.41). Another helpful finding is the "carpet tack" sign that may be elicited by lifting the adherent scale and revealing keratotic spikes. Always check inside the ears as follicular plugging in the ear is another useful sign of DLE. Symptoms may include itching, pain, burning, and tenderness.

Lupus profundus may be suspected clinically in an irregularly shaped alopecic patch that shows dyspigmentation and follicular plugging that resembles large comedones (Figs. 6.42 and 6.43).

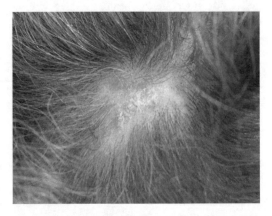

Fig. 6.39 DLE with central plugging in the center of the alopecia patch

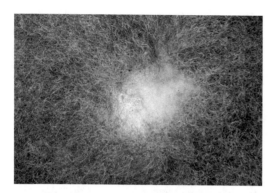

Fig. 6.40 DLE with central plugging and hypo- and hyperpigmentation

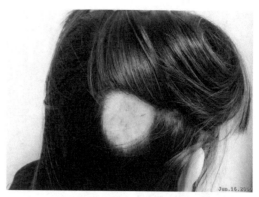

Fig. 6.42 Lupus profundus in a 30-year-old Asian woman a with solitary occipital bare patch. See Fig 6.43 for close-up details that suggest the diagnosis

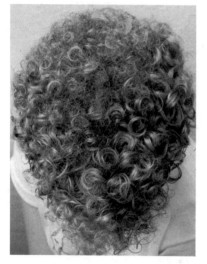

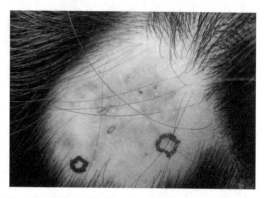

Fig. 6.43 Close-up details of lupus profundus (Fig. 6.42). Note the irregular shape of the alopecic patch, the dyspigmentation, and the follicular plugging that resembles large comedones. Biopsy sites are marked in *black*

Fig. 6.41 Same patient as in Fig. 6.40 showing increased curliness of hair overlying the patch of DLE

If DLE is treated early, the hair loss is potentially reversible. If not treated early, over half the patients will develop scarring alopecia. The end stage of DLE is clinically distinct, just as the early phase is distinct, with striking hypo- and hyperpigmentation (Fig 9.3). Dyspigmentation is not seen in the end stage of the primary cicatricial alopecias, which all look similar with large areas of total hair loss and loss of follicular ostia.

The seeming wide variation of CCLE incidence is mainly due to referral practices. Depending where physicians with a special interest in CCLE practice, patients are referred to these centers and physicians, which may be general medical clinics, and in other centers they are mainly referred to hair clinics. In the San Francisco Bay area, the incidence of CCLE seen in our hair clinic is small (Fig. 1.1) in contrast to the hair center at the University of British Columbia where CCLE accounts for 30–40% of patients with scarring alopecia.

Takeaway Pearls

> Within CCLE are three major forms: the most common is DLE, and the less common forms are lupus profundus and lupus tumidus.

> CCLE is not a primary cicatricial alopecia because in none of the three major forms is the hair follicle the target of a folliculocentric inflammatory attack.

> Hypo- and hyperpigmentation, telangiectasia, and follicular plugging in the *center* of affected patches are characteristic features of DLE, and are not typically found in the primary cicatricial alopecias.
> The "carpet tack" sign is a helpful finding in DLE.
> DLE most commonly affects the scalp, face, and ears. Always look in the ears.
> If treated early, DLE is potentially reversible.
> The end stage of DLE is clinically distinct with striking hypo- and hyperpigmentation.
> Lupus profundus may be suspected in an irregularly shaped alopecic patch with dyspigmentation and follicular plugging that resembles large comedones.

Suggested Reading

Hordinsky M. Cicatricial alopecia: discoid lupus erythematosus. Dermatol Ther. 2008;21:245–8.
Lee L. Lupus erythematosus. In: Bolognia JL, Jorizzo JL, Rapini RP, editors. Dermatology. 2nd ed. Philadelphia, PA: Mosby; 2003. p. 601–13.
Ross EK, Tan E, Shapiro J. Update on primary cicatricial alopecias. J Am Acad Dermatol. 2005;53:1–37.
Shapiro J. Cicatricial (scarring) alopecia. In: Shapiro J, editor. Hair loss: principles of diagnosis and management of alopecia. London: Martin Dunitz Ltd; 2002. p. 155–74.
Tan E, Martinka M, Ball N, et al. Primary cicatricial alopecias: clinicopathology of 112 cases. 2004;50:25–32.
Walling HW, Sontheimer RD. Cutaneous lupus erythematosus: issues in diagnosis and treatment. Am J Clin Dermatol. 2009;10:365–81.
Whiting DA. Cicatricial alopecia: clinico-pathological findings and treatment. Clin Dermatol. 2001;19:211–25.

Keratosis Follicularis Spinulosa Decalvans

Clinical Scenario

A 6-year-old boy is brought in by his parents for evaluation of hair loss. The patient has developed progressive hair loss starting in infancy. There is no family history of childhood hair loss. On exam, he has noninflammatory, flesh-colored, spiny lesions affecting hair-bearing areas including the scalp, brows, and eyelids. He also has thickening of the skin of his heels.

Making the Diagnosis

Keratosis follicularis is a rare genodermatosis that has clinical features of a scarring alopecia.

History

• Onset is in infancy.
• Family history may be present.

Exam

• Absence of follicular ostia.
• Spiny lesions affecting all hair-bearing areas.
• Hair loss of the scalp, brows, eyelashes is patchy, rarely total.
• Associated keratoderma sometimes present.
• Associated keratitis.

Discussion

The term keratosis follicularis spinulosa decalvans (*KFSD*) was first used by Siemens in 1926 who described a scarring follicular condition in 20 members of a large family. Unlike the primary cicatricial alopecias that have their onset in adults, KFSD begins in infancy with noninflammatory, keratotic, spiny lesions affecting hair-bearing areas, especially the scalp and later eyebrows, eyelids, and the dorsum of the hands and fingers. On occasion, more proximal limbs and even the trunk become involved. Associated findings include plantar keratoderma as well as various ocular changes. Photophobia and punctate corneal epithelial defects may occur due to a primary epithelial defect or as a result of irritation from distorted lashes. Rare ophthalmologic abnormalities, including cataracts and retinal detachment, have also been reported. The disease tends to progress until puberty, with patchy scarring alopecia of scalp, eyebrows, and eyelashes. Axillary and pubic hair is often thinned.

The histologic findings in KFSD have significant overlap with those of primary cicatricial alopecias with follicular-based hyperkeratosis, perifollicular and dermal inflammation, fibrotic tracts, and distorted follicles.

Family studies suggest an X-linked dominant inheritance pattern, with men often more severely affected than women. The mutated gene encoding the spermidine/spermine $N(1)$-acetyltransferase (SSAT) has been localized to Xp22.13-p22.2. However, clinical heterogeneity is likely as there has been identification of pedigrees unlinked to this region as well as rare instances of male-to-male transmission suggesting an autosomal dominant form.

In general, treatment of KFSD is unsuccessful in halting the progression of disease, especially the alopecia; however, there are isolated reports of improvement in photophobia with oral vitamin A, as well as conflicting reports of the results of dapsone and oral retinoids.

A variant of KFSD that has a more persistent pustular course has been called *folliculitis spinulosa decalvans*. Unlike KFSD, patients with *folliculitis spinulosa decalvans* often have symptoms of severe inflammation that go beyond puberty. In addition, the inheritance appears to be autosomal dominant rather than X-linked recessive. Treatment response to isotretinoin has been unsuccessful. Laser-assisted hair removal was successful in reducing the recalcitrant inflammation and pain in a 23-year-old Caucasian male, who appreciated and felt liberated by the subsequent absence of pain and inflammation (Fig. 6.44).

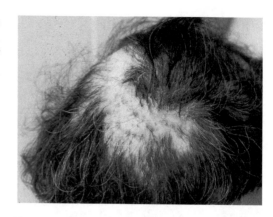

Fig. 6.44 23-year-old Caucasian male with folliculitis spinulosa decalvans. Note the extensive hair loss with perifollicular scaling, crusting, erythema, and tufting. His inflamed scalp was constantly painful and unresponsive to systemic antibiotics and topical anti-inflammatory agents. He had keratosis pilaris on his arms and thighs, but was otherwise healthy. He agreed to have permanent hair removal with the EpiLaser to reduce the scalp inflammation. The hair removal proved successful, and his life was totally changed when the chronic scalp discomfort was removed

Suggested Reading

Castori M, Covaciu C, Paradisi M, et al. Clinical and genetic heterogeneity in keratosis follicularis spinulosa decalvans. Eur J Med Genet. 2009;52:53–8.

Chui CT, Berger TG, Price VH, et al. Recalcitrant scarring follicular disorders treated by laser-assisted hair removal: a preliminary report. Dermatol Surg. 1999;25:34–7.

Hallai N, Thompson I, Williams P, et al. Folliculitis spinulosa decalvans: failure to respond to oral isotretinoin. J Eur Acad Dermatol Venereol. 2006;20:223–4.

Oosterwijk JC, Nelen M, van Zandvoort PM, et al. Linkage analysis of keratosis follicularis spinulosa decalvans, and regional assignment to human chromosome Xp21.2-p22.2. Am J Hum Genet. 1992;50:801–7.

Oranje AP, van Osch LD, Oosterwijk JC. Keratosis pilaris atrophicans. One heterogeneous disease or a symptom in different clinical entities? Arch Dermatol. 1994;130:469–75.

Predominantly Neutrophilic Group

Vera Price and Paradi Mirmirani

The predominantly neutrophilic group of primary cicatricial alopecias includes folliculitis decalvans and tufted folliculitis. Clinically, the affected areas are much more inflamed than the lymphocytic cicatricial alopecias with crusting, pustules, draining, and erythema. There is usually considerable pain, tenderness, and itching. Histologically in the early stages, the inflammatory infiltrate consists predominantly of neutrophils. However, the infiltrate does not remain neutrophilic but rather becomes plasma-cell rich. What other histologic features can be used as clues to a neutrophilic cicatricial alopecia that is no longer predominantly neutrophilic? Scan the scalp biopsy with low-power light microscopy: the presence of four or more fused follicles, and dense interfollicular inflammation and fibrosis are diagnostically useful (see Chap. 3).

Folliculitis Decalvans

Clinical Scenario

A 30-year-old Caucasian man seeks treatment for hair loss of 1 year's duration. He has had "dandruff" for many years and then developed "irritated bumps" on his scalp for which he used antidandruff shampoos. The bumps and dandruff have persisted, and now he has noticed hair loss, tenderness, "oozing," and bloody crusting on the scalp and staining on his pillows. The patient is otherwise healthy. On exam, he has impressive patchy areas of hair loss with absent follicular markings throughout the scalp. Erythema, crusting, and tufted follicles rim the bare patches (Fig. 7.1) and there is scaling throughout the scalp. A few pustules are present. Pull test yields one anagen and two telogen hairs (Pull test: 1/3). Eyebrows, eyelashes, and fingernails are normal. Oral mucous membranes are clear and remainder of his skin exam is unremarkable. A 4-mm scalp biopsy is taken from the edge of a bare patch, and pustules are cultured for bacteria and fungi.

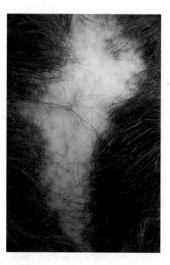

Fig. 7.1 Folliculitis decalvans with central loss of hair, absent follicular ostia, and acute activity with erythema, crusting, pustules, and hair tufts at the margins

V. Price and P. Mirmirani (eds.), *Cicatricial Alopecia: An Approach to Diagnosis and Management*, DOI 10.1007/978-1-4419-8399-2_7, © Springer Science+Business Media, LLC 2011

Making the Diagnosis

History

- Symptoms include scalp pain, itching, and burning
- Bloody crusting noted on the scalp and staining of his pillows
- Many year history of seborrheic dermatitis

Physical Exam

- Impressive patches of hair loss with erythema, crusting, pustules, and tufted follicles mainly around the outer rim of the bare patches
- Loss of follicular markings
- Diffuse scaling
- Positive anagen pull test (1/3)
- Brows, lashes, nails, and skin are unaffected

Laboratory Testing

- Bacterial culture: Mild to moderate growth of *Staphylococcus aureus*
- Fungal culture: negative

Scalp Biopsy

- Decreased numbers of follicles and a moderate neutrophilic and plasmacytic perifollicular infiltrate, with moderate interfollicular inflammation and scarred fibrous tracts. Compound follicles with four and five fused follicles

The clinical and histologic features support a diagnosis of folliculitis decalvans.

Discussion

Folliculitis decalvans along with tufted folliculitis represent the primary cicatricial alopecias with a suppurative phase. Decalvans is a term derived from the Latin meaning "making bald"; Brocq et al. in 1905 used the term folliculitis decalvans (FD) to describe a rare form of scalp folliculitis that led to permanent or scarring alopecia. Although extensive epidemiologic studies are not available, the frequency of FD is about 11% of all cicatricial alopecia cases (Fig. 1.1). Onset is in young and middle-aged adults, and men and women are both affected.

Patients frequently present with scalp pain, itching, and bloody crusting. They may be aware of staining on their pillows. The course is usually chronic with crops of pustules, much inflammation, and eventually patchy hair loss. With progression, the bare patches may coalesce to involve large areas of the scalp, often on the vertex and occipital region. A typical bare, shiny scarred area shows absence of follicular ostia, while at the margins there is bright erythema, scaling, crusting, and tufting (Figs. 7.1–7.3). Unlike dissecting cellulitis, sinus tract formation is not a feature of folliculitis decalvans.

Tufted follicles are commonly seen around areas of folliculitis decalvans. The "hair bumps" that patients describe on their scalp are the thick hair tufts. Many clinicians consider tufted folliculitis a mild variant of folliculitis decalvans because the histopathology of the two conditions is indistinguishable. We concur with these observations. However, in some patients, tufted follicles are the predominant finding with only one or more small affected areas, and hair loss is notably minimal. In some of these patients, the tufted follicles are shed and the areas are subsequently difficult to find. We favor retaining the designation tufted folliculitis as a separate entity because of the different clinical presentation (affected areas are small and hair loss is minimal) and better prognosis in these patients (see

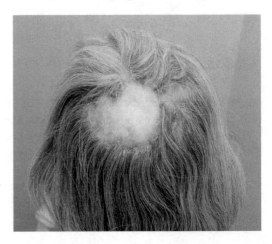

Fig. 7.2 Folliculitis decalvans with central loss of hair, loss of follicular ostia, and acute inflammation at margins with erythema and crusting

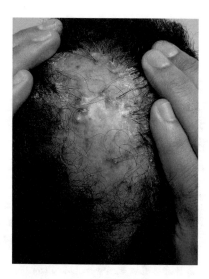

Fig. 7.3 Folliculitis decalvans with central loss of hair, absent follicular ostia, and erythema, pustules, and hair tufts at the margins

section below: Tufted Folliculitis). However, if the affected areas enlarge into large areas of hair loss, we change the designation to folliculitis decalvans.

Repeated cultures and sensitivities are essential to guide selection of appropriate antimicrobial agents. The first choice for bacterial cultures are fresh pustules; if no pustules are present, lift up a site of scalp crusting and culture the underlying skin, or culture a small deep scalp biopsy, or culture hair bulbs obtained in a pull test. A nasal swab is done to see if the patient is a carrier of *S. aureus*. If the inflammation is notably difficult to control, take repeated cultures and suspect an anaerobic presence (uncommon), and inquire about household pets (dogs). If severe itching suddenly becomes a predominant symptom, a fungal infection may be superimposed on the underlying scarring alopecia: inquire about contact with children with tinea capitis.

S. aureus is the most commonly cultured pathogen from the scalp of patients with folliculitis decalvans and is thought to play a role in pathogenesis. However, other pathogens may also be cultured. It has been proposed that the pathogenesis of folliculitis decalvans may involve an aberrant host response to microbial organisms. Such organisms may act as "superantigens" by binding to Major Histocompatibility Complex class II molecules but may escape detection by

the host immune system. However, patients with folliculitis decalvans do not have evidence of bacterial infection elsewhere on the skin, nor do they have any evidence of immune deficiency. In this respect, this may be similar to healthy athletes who have chronic furunculosis.

Appropriate and long-term antimicrobial therapy directed at the predominant pathogen is needed to minimize the symptoms and signs of folliculitis decalvans. Repeated culture of pustules is needed to guide your choice of antimicrobial agents, and this may change over time. See Chap. 4 for a detailed discussion of treatment.

Additional Figures (Figs. 7.4–7.9)

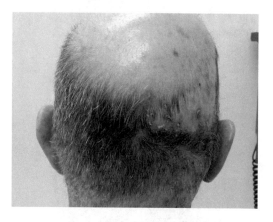

Fig. 7.4 Folliculitis decalvans demonstrating the folliculocentric aspect of primary cicatricial alopecia. In this bald man, only the hair-bearing occipital scalp is active and inflamed with pustules and crusting, and the bald scalp is spared

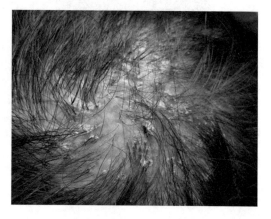

Fig. 7.5 Folliculitis decalvans with erythema, crusting, pustules, and hair tufts

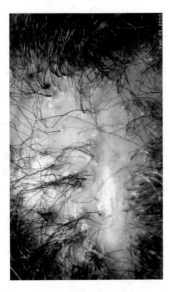

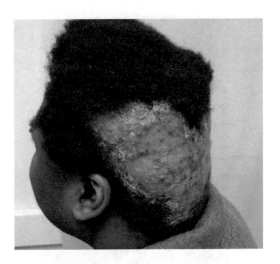

Fig. 7.8 Folliculitis decalvans with extensive scarring and erythema, loss of follicular ostia, and active crusting at margins

Fig. 7.6 Folliculitis decalvans with erythema, crusting, pustules, and hair tufts

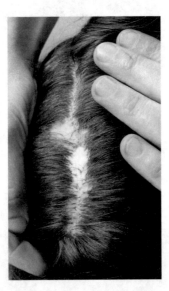

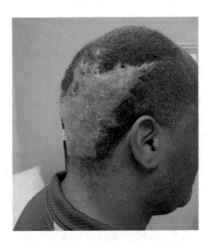

Fig. 7.9 Folliculitis decalvans, late stage, with extensive keloidal scarring and erythema

Fig. 7.7 Folliculitis decalvans, largely late stage and inactive, with faint erythema at margins. Note the patient's thick hair

Takeaway Pearls

> Impressive patches of hair loss with erythema, crusting, pustules, and tufted follicles around the rim

> Vertex and occipital scalp often favored sites

> Severe pain, discomfort, or itching

> Bloody crusting on the scalp and pillows

> Absence of follicular ostia

> Many year history of seborrheic dermatitis not uncommon

> Repeated cultures and sensitivities are essential to guide selection of appropriate antimicrobial agents

> Most common pathogen cultured from the scalp is *S. aureus*

> If the inflammation is notably difficult to control, take repeated cultures, and suspect an anaerobic presence (uncommon). Inquire about household pets (dogs), and the patient's occupation and work environment

> If severe itching suddenly becomes a predominant symptom, a fungal infection may be superimposed on the underlying scarring alopecia. Inquire about contact with children

Suggested Reading

Annessi G. Tufted folliculitis of the scalp: a distinctive clinicohistological variant of follicultis decalvans. Br J Dermatol. 1998;138:799–805.

Brocq L, Reglet J, Ayrignaq J. Recherches sur l'alopecie atrophicante. Ann Dermatol Syphil. 1905:6:1–32.

Brooke RC, Griffths CE. Folliculitis decalvans. Clin Exp Dermatol. 2001;26:120–2.

Chandrawansa PH, Giam Y. Folliculitis decalvans – a retrospective study in a tertiary referred center, over five years. Singapore Med J. 2003;44:84–7.

Dawber RPR, Fenton DA. Cicatricial alopecia. In: Dawber R, editor. Diseases of the hair and scalp. 3rd ed. Oxford: Blackwell; 1997. p. 370–96.

Powell J, Dawber RPR. Successful treatment regime for folliculitis decalvans despite uncertainty of all etiological factors. Br J Dermatol. 2001;143:195–7.

Powell JJ, Dawber RP, Gatter K. Folliculitis decalvans including tufted folliculitis: clinical histological
and therapeutic findings. Br J Dermatol. 1999;140:328–33.

Ross EK, Tan E, Shapiro J. Update on primary cicatricial alopecias. J Am Acad Dermatol. 2005;53:1–37.

Sperling LC, Solomon AR, Whiting DA. A new look at scarring alopecia. Arch Dermatol. 2000;136:235–42.

Tan E, Martinka M, Ball N, et al. Primary cicatricial alopecias: clinicopathology of 112 cases. J Am Acad Dermatol. 2004:50:25–32.

Whiting DA. Cicatricial alopecia: clinico-pathological findings and treatment. Clin Dermatol 2001:19:211–15.

Tufted Folliculitis

Clinical Scenario

A 42-year-old Caucasian man presents to the clinic with a solitary patch of hair loss associated with itching and pain and he describes feeling "scalp bumps" in the area. His health is good. He is using an antidandruff shampoo and has been given oral antibiotics in the past, both of which help to decrease the severity of his symptoms. On exam, the patient has a solitary 3 × 2 cm area of hair loss at the vertex with crusting, pustules, erythema, decreased follicular ostia, and prominent thick tufted hairs around the margins (Fig. 7.10). Pull test yields one anagen and one telogen hair (Pull test: 1/2). A 4-mm scalp biopsy and bacterial cultures are taken.

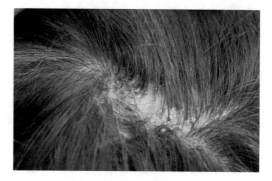

Fig. 7.10 Tufted folliculitis. Small solitary patch of hair loss with crusting, erythema, decreased follicular ostia and prominent hair tufts

Making the Diagnosis

History

- Symptoms of itching, pain, and "scalp bumps"

Physical Exam

- Small area of hair loss with erythema, crusting, pustules, and tufted hairs

Laboratory Testing

- Culture: Moderate growth of *S. aureus*

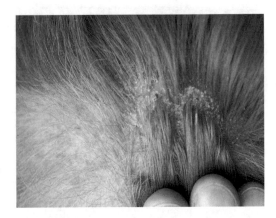

Fig. 7.11 Tufted folliculitis with impressive thick hair tufts, scaling, crusting, erythema, and minimal hair loss

Biopsy

- Moderate neutrophilic and plasmacytic infiltrate around the infundibulum; numerous compound follicles with four and five fused follicles

  The clinical and histological findings support the diagnosis of tufted folliculitis.

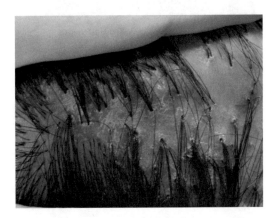

Fig. 7.12 Tufted folliculitis. Thick tufts appear like cords resembling synthetic implants

Discussion

The term tufted folliculitis is used to describe a primary cicatricial alopecia in which tufts of hair are the cardinal and prominent feature surrounding relatively small patches of hair loss. Usually there are only a few affected areas on the scalp which also show erythema, scaling, crusting, and pustules. The thick hair tufts or bundles each contain four or more hairs all exiting the scalp from a single orifice and often resemble cords or synthetic implants (Figs. 7.11–7.13). The areas are itchy and painful, and the "hair bumps" that patients describe on their scalp are the thick hair tufts.

As with FD, *S. aureus* is the most common pathogen cultured. These patients are otherwise healthy and have no known immune deficiency.

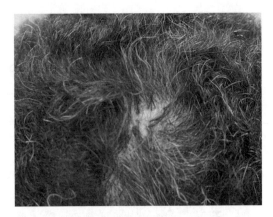

Fig 7.13 Tufted folliculitis. Small patch of hair loss with prominent hair tufts

Fig 7.14 Designation of tufted folliculitis arbitrarily changed to folliculitis decalvans when hair loss becomes extensive

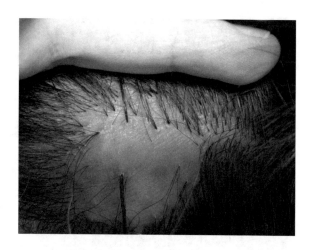

Management includes repeated cultures and sensitivities of pustules. Treatment of tufted folliculitis is outlined in Chap. 4.

Many clinicians consider tufted folliculitis as a mild variant of folliculitis decalvans because the histopathology of the two conditions is indistinguishable, and *S. aureus* is usually cultured from the lesions in both. We concur with these observations. However, in some patients, tufted follicles are the predominant finding in one or more small areas, and hair loss is notably minimal. In some of these patients, the tufted follicles disappear, most probably are shed, and the areas are subsequently difficult to locate. In others, the affected areas remain small with prominent tufted follicles and minimal hair loss. We favor retaining the designation tufted folliculitis as a separate entity because of the different clinical presentation (affected areas are small and hair loss is minimal) and better prognosis in these patients. This is a useful concept for the clinician managing such a patient. In contrast, in some patients, the affected areas enlarge into large areas of hair loss; we then change the designation to folliculitis decalvans (Fig. 7.14). Whether one is a "lumper" or a "splitter," we anticipate that in future molecular markers will indicate which pathway the tufted folliculitis will follow.

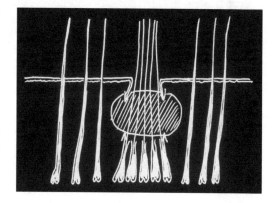

Fig. 7.15 Schematic drawing of formation of a hair tuft. Courtesy of VH Price, MD

Tufted follicles form when the epithelial walls of adjacent follicles are destroyed by intense inflammation at the level of the infundibulum. The indestructible keratin fibers (hairs) fall together and exit as a tuft in a large common infundibulum (Fig. 7.15).

It should be noted that *tufted follicles* may be seen in the late stage of any primary cicatricial alopecia and in the late stage of secondary cicatricial alopecias including those due to inflammatory dermatoses, physical and chemical injury, infections, and neoplasms.

Takeaway Pearls

> Clinically: itching, pain, and "scalp bumps"
> One or more small areas of hair loss with erythema, crusting, pustules, and prominent hair tufts
> Hair loss is minimal
> Hair tufts contain four or more hairs and resemble cords or synthetic implants
> Most common pathogen cultured from the scalp is *S. aureus*
> We favor retaining the designation tufted folliculitis as a separate entity from folliculitis decalvans because the clinical presentation is milder and the prognosis may be better. Affected areas are small and hair loss is minimal; in some patients the tufted follicles are shed and areas are difficult to find.

> If areas of hair loss enlarge, we arbitrarily change the designation to folliculitis decalvans

Suggested Reading

Annessi G. Tufted folliculitis of the scalp: a distinctive clinicohistological variant of folliculitis decalvans. Br J Dermatol. 1998;138:799–805.

Dawber RPR, Fenton DA. Cicatricial alopecia. In: Dawber R, editor. Diseases of the hair and scalp. 3rd ed. Oxford: Blackwell; 1997. p. 370–96.

Ross EK, Tan E, Shapiro J. Update on primary cicatricial alopecias. J Am Acad Dermatol. 2005;53:1–37.

Tan E, Martinka M, Ball N, et al. Primary cicatricial alopecias: clinicopathology of 112 cases. J Am Acad Dermatol. 2004;50:25–32.

Whiting DA. Cicatricial alopecia: clinico-pathological findings and treatment. Clinics Dermatol. 2001;19: 211–25.

Mixed Group

8

Vera Price and Paradi Mirmirani

The inflammation in dissecting cellulitis and folliculitis keloidalis is secondary to follicular rupture and the release of sebaceous and keratinous material and hair keratin fragments. The latter incite an intense inflammatory response. The inflammation is initially neutrophilic and later mixed with lymphocytes, plasma cells, and foreign body giant cells; granulomas may form around the hair keratin fragments. Sinus tract formation is prominent in dissecting cellulitis and rarely found in folliculitis keloidalis. Unlike folliculitis decalvans and tufted folliculitis in which *Staphylococcus aureus* is usually cultured, in the mixed group, bacterial pathogens are not usually found. Dissecting cellulitis is considered part of the follicular occlusion triad, which includes acne conglobata and hidradenitis suppurativa. The pathogenesis of folliculitis keloidalis is not well understood.

Dissecting Cellulitis

Clinical Scenario

A 22-year-old African-American reports hair loss and ongoing "boils" on his scalp since his teens. Oral antibiotics help only briefly. He first developed "boils" above his hairline at the back of his scalp in his late teens. The hair loss and boils have progressed to involve most of his scalp, and he recently noticed red bumps under his arms. The patient is otherwise healthy and is not taking any medications. On exam, he has confluent boggy sinus tracts on his scalp with purulent drainage and crusting. He has mild facial acne and a few erythematous nodules in both axillae with mild cervical lymphadenopathy. His eyebrows, eyelashes, and nails are normal.

Making the Diagnosis

- Dissecting cellulitis presents most frequently in young dark-skinned men. Painful nodules and interconnecting sinus tracts on the scalp with purulent drainage, crusting, and patchy alopecia are characteristic

History

- Symptoms started in the teens
- Painful scalp "boils" or nodules with purulent drainage

Exam

- Nodules on the scalp with interconnecting sinus tracts
- Purulent drainage and crusting
- Also has hidradenitis suppurativa but only mild acne
- Brows, lashes, nails unaffected

V. Price and P. Mirmirani (eds.), *Cicatricial Alopecia: An Approach to Diagnosis and Management*,
DOI 10.1007/978-1-4419-8399-2_8, © Springer Science+Business Media, LLC 2011

Laboratory Testing

- Bacterial culture grew coagulase-negative *Staphyloccocus*
- Fungal culture was negative

Scalp Biopsy

- Biopsy shows marked reduction in follicular density with a mixed infiltrate of neutrophils, histiocytes, lymphocytes, and plasmacytes in the interfollicular dermis. Extensive coarse fibrosis is present both in the perifollicular adventitial dermis and the reticular dermis.

The clinical findings and histology support the diagnosis of dissecting cellulitis.

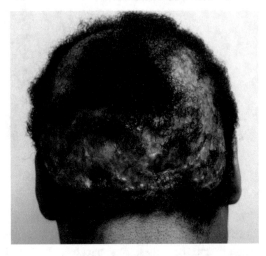

Fig. 8.1 Dissecting cellulitis in 31-year-old man with nodules, sinus tracts, and extensive scarring and hair loss

Discussion

Dissecting cellulitis is an uncommon but readily recognized chronic inflammatory disease of scalp hair follicles. It is also known as dissecting folliculitis or perifolliculitis capitis abscedens et suffodiens. Multiple painful fluctuant nodules, interconnecting sinus tracts, and purulent drainage are characteristic. It is seen primarily in dark-skinned men in the second to fourth decade. It frequently begins in the occipital scalp and vertex, although any region of the scalp may be involved, and extensive boggy nodules and sinus tracts may be present over large areas of the scalp (Fig. 8.1). The condition tends to be chronic and progressive and ultimately leads to scarring and extensive hair loss (Fig. 8.2).

Dissecting cellulitis is considered part of the follicular occlusion triad that includes acne conglobata and hidradenitis suppurativa. In some patients, only the scalp hair follicles are affected. As a follicular occlusion disorder, a defect in follicular keratinization results in poral obstruction, and sebaceous and keratinous material accumulate within pilosebaceous units. Ultimately, the follicles burst resulting in an intense inflammatory neutrophilic reaction with sinus tract formation. It has been suggested that the pathogenesis of dissecting cellulitis may involve an abnormal host

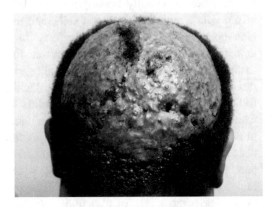

Fig. 8.2 Dissecting cellulitis in 26-year-old man with extensive scarring and hair loss. Note folliculitis keloidalis at nape. With permission: Fu JM and Price VH. Cicatricial alopecia. JDermatol Nurses' Association. 2010;2:1–5

response to bacterial antigens. However, patients with dissecting cellulitis have no evidence of immune deficiency or presence of infection at other skin sites. The drainage or pus may be sterile or grow *Propionibacterium acnes* or coagulase-negative *Staphylococcus*. Less frequently pathogenic bacteria such as *Staph. aureus* and *proteus* are cultured.

Tinea capitis is in the differential diagnosis, and in addition to a scalp biopsy, a fungal culture may be included in the workup. There may be a family history of acne or hidradenitis suppurativa.

Treatment of dissecting cellulitis is unsatisfactory in terms of permanent arrest of the condition and full hair regrowth. Oral antibiotics and isot-retinoin are used with variable success in decreasing the inflammation, but prolonged or continuous treatment is usually required. In patients with a predominant organism, antibiotics should be directed at eradication of that organism. In patients without a predominant organism, isotretinion may be helpful; the starting dose of isotretinoin must be small (10–20 mg per day) to avoid exacerbating the inflammation. However, relapses are frequent upon discontinuation of the medication, and treatment is invariably long-term. We have seen partial hair regrowth if the condition is treated early, especially in lighter-skinned men (Fig. 8.3).

Recently, several reports have shown favorable response to antitumor necrosis factor (TNF) therapy in hidradenitis suppurativa. Infliximab, which has shown promise for treatment of hidradenitis suppurativa, has been used successfully in dissecting cellulitis. We have also had success in controlling the inflammation and purulent drainage with infliximab in a patient who failed previous therapies (Fig. 8.4a, b). Adalimumab, another anti-TNF monoclonal antibody, was effective in controlling the inflammation in three patients with dissecting cellulitis. In the reported cases and in our own observations, anti-TNF therapy effectively controls the inflammation in dissecting cellulitis, but relapses are common when the drugs are discontinued, and the underlying sinus tracts are not altered. Long-term medical treatment combined with surgical drainage and resection of affected areas are often needed in dissecting cellulitis.

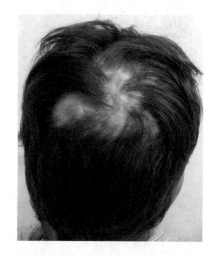

Fig. 8.3 Dissecting cellulitis in a Caucasian man with boggy nodules and sinus tracts. Note the partial hair regrowth

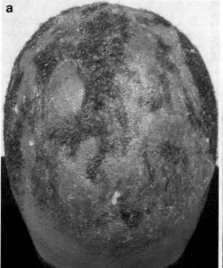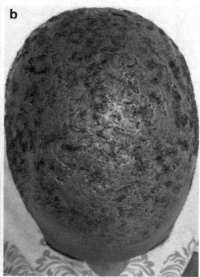

Fig. 8.4 (**a**) Dissecting cellulitis with boggy nodules, purulent drainage, crusting, and sinus tracts. (**b**) Same patient with dissecting cellulitis after successful response to infliximab and sulphamethoxazole-trimethoprim DS for 1 year. Patient had failed therapy with oral and topical antibiotics, prednisone, isotretinoin, etanercept, and intralesional triamcinolone acetonide

Additional Figures (Figs. 8.5 and 8.6)

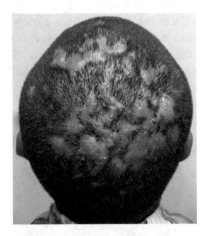

Fig. 8.5 Dissecting cellulitis

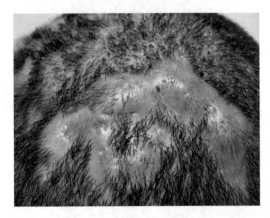

Fig. 8.6 Close up of dissecting cellulitis

Takeaway Pearls

> Seen most frequently in young dark-skinned men

> Multiple painful fluctuant nodules, interconnecting sinus tracts, and purulent drainage are characteristic

> Drainage or pus often sterile, but bacterial superinfection may occur

> If the condition is treated and arrested early, the hair loss may be partially reversible

> Generally chronic and progressive, leads to scarring and extensive hair loss

---

> Consider tinea capitis in the differential diagnosis and consider sending a fungal culture as part of the work up

> Long-term medical treatment combined with surgical drainage and resection of affected areas is often needed

> Dissecting cellulitis is considered part of the follicular occlusion triad that includes acne conglobata and hidradenitis suppurativa

Suggested Reading

Adams DR, Yankura JA, Fogelberg AC, et al. Treatment of hidradenitis suppurativa with etanercept. JAMA. 2010;146:501–4.

Brandt HR, Malheiros AP, Teixeira MG, et al. Perifolliculitis capitis abscedens et suffodiens successfully controlled with infliximab. Br J Dermatol. 2008;159:506–7.

Grant A, Gonzalez T, Montgomery MO, et al. Infliximab therapy for patients with moderate to severe hidradenitis suppurativa: a randomized, double-blind, placebo-controlled crossover trial. J Am Acad Dermatol. 2010;62:205–17.

Lebwohl B, Sapadin AN. Infliximab for the treatment of hidradenitis suppurativa. J Am Acad Dermatol. 2003;49:S275–6.

Mekkes JR, Bos JD. Long-term efficacy of a single course of infliximab in hidradenitis suppurativa. Br J Dermatol. 2008;158:370–4.

Navarini. AA, Trueb, RM. 3 cases of dissecting cellulitis of the scalp treated with adalimumab. Arch Dermatol. 2010;146:517–20.

Ross EK, Tan E, Shapiro J. Update on primary cicatricial alopecias. J Am Acad Dermatol. 2005;53:1–37.

Tan E, Martinka M, Ball N, et al. Primary cicatricial alopecias: Clinicopathology of 112 cases. J Am Acad Dermatol. 2004;50:25–32.

Whiting DA. Cicatricial alopecia: clinico-pathological findings and treatment. Clinics Dermatol. 2001;19:211–25.

Folliculitis Keloidalis

Clinical Scenario

A 25-year-old African-American man presents in clinic with a complaint of "bumps" on the back of his scalp, which have been present since age

16 and have become progressively larger over time. He has some discomfort and itching in the affected area and is occasionally able to express pus from the bumps. He wears his hair shaved or clipped short. On exam, there are multiple small, firm, flesh-colored papules and nodules in the nuchal and lower occipital area. The larger papules and nodules are hairless.

Making the Diagnosis

History

- The patient is a young dark-skinned male who has a history of shaving or clipping his hair short

Physical Exam

- Small papules and nodules are predominantly in the nuchal and lower occipital area

Biopsy

- A mixed inflammatory perifollicular infiltrate with neutrophils, lymphocytes, and plasma cells at the level of the isthmus with loss of sebaceous glands. Few "naked" hair fragments in the dermis

The clinical and histologic findings support a diagnosis of folliculitis keloidalis.

Discussion

Synonyms for this disorder include acne keloidalis and acne keloidalis nuchae. We prefer to use the term folliculitis keloidalis (FK) as "acne" is a misnomer, and the lesions are not always limited to the nuchal area of the scalp.

The classification of FK is not settled. As with dissecting cellulitis, we consider FK secondary to rupture of a hair follicle, and the marked inflammation and granulomatous reaction due to

released sebaceous material and extruded hair shaft fragments.

FK predominantly affects the nuchal area of young men of African or other dark-skinned ancestry, and rarely in dark-skinned women and Caucasians. The disorder tends to occur in younger patients, and lesions may appear as early as the teens. In early stages, small, flesh-colored, firm papules and pustules occur over the nuchal region and occipital scalp (Fig. 8.7–8.9). If treated aggressively, the lesions may resolve and hair loss may not be permanent. However, if FK is untreated or if it progresses, the small papules persist, may enlarge and fuse to form nodules or keloidal plaques; sinus tract formation is largely absent. Tufted hairs and pustules are often noted at the periphery of the plaques. Symptoms range from minimal to moderate itching, discomfort, or pain. FK may coexist with other forms of cicatricial alopecia including folliculitis decalvans and dissecting cellulitis (Fig. 8.2).

The cause of FK is unclear. It has been ascribed to trauma, often from a razor or hair clippers, shirt collars, and short haircuts, but none of these is established. In predisposed patients, follicular rupture may initiate an intense neutrophilic inflammatory response; degenerating hair fragments contribute to the intense and widespread dermal inflammation and fibrosis. Some view

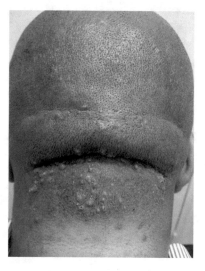

Fig. 8.7 Folliculitis keloidalis with papules and nodules in the nuchal and lower occipital area

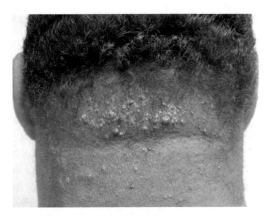

Fig. 8.8 Folliculitis keloidalis with papules in nuchal area

folliculocentric events. Genetic predisposition undoubtedly plays a role.

Histopathological findings vary depending on the stage of the process. In early disease, after rupture of a follicle, the inflammation is primarily neutrophilic, with dense dermal inflammation and fibrosis. In older lesions, the inflammation is mixed and includes neutrophils, plasma cells, and foreign body giant cells. Sebaceous glands are destroyed, and residual hair fragments elicit a granulomatous reaction.

The treatment of FK depends on the stage of the condition (see Chap. 4).

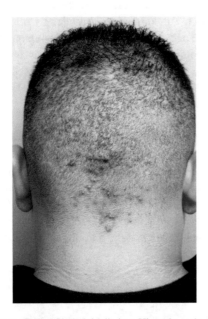

Fig. 8.9 Folliculitis keloidalis in a Hispanic male. Note the small flesh-colored papules and larger keloidal plaques in the occipital area

FK as a primary cicatricial alopecia based on the histopathologic characteristics (perifollicular inflammation at the level of the isthmus and lower infundibulum, loss of sebaceous glands, inflamed and destroyed follicles, residual naked hair fragments). We view these findings as secondary to the follicular rupture, rather than as primary

> **Takeaway Pearls**
>
> › Typical patient is a young dark-skinned male who has a history of shaving or clipping his hair short
> › Small papules and nodules are predominantly in the nuchal area and lower occipital area
> › FK may coexist with other forms of cicatricial alopecia including folliculitis decalvans and dissecting cellulitis

Suggested Reading

Khumalo NP, Jessop S, Gumedze F, et al. Hairdressing is associated with scalp disease in African schoolchildren. Br J Dermatol. 2007;157:106–10.

Khumalo NP, Jessop S, Gumedze F, et al. Hairdressing and the prevalence of scalp disease in African adults. Br J Dermatol. 2007;157:981–8.

Sperling LC, Homoky C, Pratt L, et al. Acne keloidalis is a form of primary scarring alopecia. Arch Dermatol. 2000;136:479–84.

Ross EK, Tan E, Shapiro J. Update on primary cicatricial alopecias. J Am Acad Dermatol. 2005;53:1–37.

Tan E, Martinka M, Ball N, et al. Primary cicatricial alopecias: clinicopathology of 112 cases. J Am Acad Dermatol. 2004;50:25–32.

Whiting DA. Cicatricial alopecia: clinico-pathological findings and treatment. Clin Dermatol. 2001;19:211–25.

End Stage Nonspecific Group

Vera Price and Paradi Mirmirani

9

Clinical Scenario

A 45-year-old man presents with extensive asymptomatic hair loss affecting most of the top of his scalp. Ten years earlier, he was seen by a dermatologist for patchy hair loss and he remembers having much pain and itching. Scalp biopsy at that time showed lichen planopilaris. His treatment included hydroxychloroquine 200 mg twice daily and intralesional triamcinolone acetonide. He was lost to follow up until his current visit. Scalp examination at the present time shows complete, confluent hair loss over the entire top of his scalp with absence of follicular markings and absence of any clinical inflammation (Fig. 9.1). Currently, there is no clinical clue regarding the diagnosis of his original patchy hair loss. A scalp biopsy is taken.

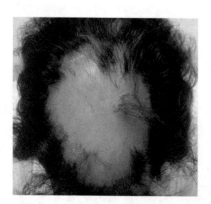

Fig. 9.1 End-stage, nonspecific cicatricial alopecia, not further classifiable. Note absent inflammation and loss of follicular ostia. Ten years earlier the patient had a diagnosis of LPP

Making the Diagnosis

History

- Patient remembers his hair loss 10 years ago when it was patchy, painful, and itchy
- He is now asymptomatic
- Bare areas have gradually merged to form one large bare area on the top of the scalp

Exam

- Confluent hair loss over entire frontal/parietal scalp
- Loss of follicular markings: scalp looks like a smooth skating rink
- Absence of any clinical inflammation

Scalp Biopsy

- Few hair follicles, minimal infiltrate, many scarred fibrous tracts
- Absent sebaceous glands

Discussion

The clinical scenario demonstrates that LPP in the acute stage is clinically distinct, but in the late stage, the distinguishing features are no

V. Price and P. Mirmirani (eds.), *Cicatricial Alopecia: An Approach to Diagnosis and Management,*
DOI 10.1007/978-1-4419-8399-2_9, © Springer Science+Business Media, LLC 2011

longer present and a specific diagnosis can no longer be made.

The acute stage of the primary cicatricial alopecias is clinically distinct and a tentative diagnosis can usually be made based on the location, pattern, morphology, and inflammatory features. The experienced clinician, who has seen many patients with cicatricial alopecia, can usually diagnose untreated LPP, FFA, PPB, CCCA, FD and distinguish them clinically from DLE with a high degree of accuracy. However, over time, or with treatment, these clinical aspects become less distinct. Finally, in the late or end stage of these diseases, the characteristic features are no longer present, and the various entities become clinically indistinguishable with bare patches that may have coalesced into large bare areas, without follicular ostia, and without inflammation (Figs. 9.1–9.3). DLE is the exception: it can usually be distinguished clinically in the acute stage from the primary lymphocytic cicatricial alopecias, as well as in the late or end stage, which is recognized by the hypo- and hyperpigmentation of the scalp, and follicular plugging and hypo- and hyperpigmentation in the ears (Fig. 9.4).

A note of caution: be careful not to misdiagnose a patient with acute stage PPB or CCCA as having end stage disease because of the absence of symptoms or signs. Patients with PPB and CCCA often have no overt symptoms and signs, even in the acute stage of their disease. A history of continued spreading of their hair loss is indication for a scalp biopsy. In these patients, it is useful to record the size of the affected area(s) with photography, or measurements, if practical, because spreading of the hair loss and the extent of the inflammatory infiltrate (as seen on scalp biopsy) are the only two indicators of ongoing activity and signal the need for treatment. A moderate or dense lymphocytic infiltrate is indication for systemic treatment.

As mentioned in Chap. 6: Pseudopelade (Brocq), we recommend that readers abandon using the term "pseudopelade" to describe end-stage cicatricial alopecia. Instead, the preferred terminology to describe the late or burned out stage of any cicatricial alopecia is "end-stage, nonspecific cicatricial alopecia" when clinical

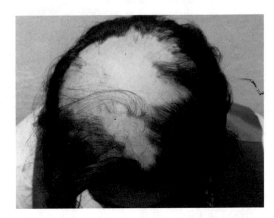

Fig. 9.2 End-stage, nonspecific cicatricial alopecia, not further classifiable. Note absent inflammation and loss of follicular ostia. Ten years earlier the patient had a diagnosis of PPB. With permission: Fu JM, Price VH. Cicatricial alopecia. J Dermatol Nurses' Assoc. 2010;2:1–5

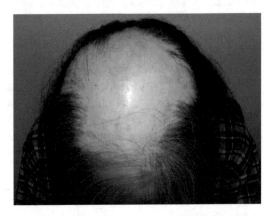

Fig. 9.3 End stage, nonspecific cicatricial alopecia, not further classifiable. Note absent inflammation and loss of follicular ostia. Ten years earlier the patient had a diagnosis of folliculitis decalvans

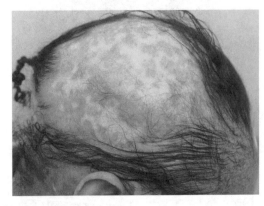

Fig. 9.4 End-stage DLE is recognizable by the hypo- and hyperpigmentation on the scalp and in the ears

Table 9.1 Clinical features that help to distinguish PPB, LPP, CCCA, AA

	PPB	LPP	CCCA	AA
Distribution: central, symmetrical	No	No	Yes	No
Very symptomatic	No	Yes	No	No
Perifollicular erythema/scaling	No	Yes	No	No
Loss of follicular ostia	Yes	Yes	Yes	No
Color of affected patches	White	Flesh color	Flesh color	Peach color

differentiation is no longer possible and histology shows sparse follicles, dermal fibrosis, scarred fibrous tracts, and loss of sebaceous glands. The term pseudopelade (Brocq) (PPB) should be used to describe the primary lymphocytic cicatricial alopecia. Table 9.1 helps distinguish the clinical features of PPB, LPP, CCCA, and alopecia areata (AA).

Takeaway Pearls

> Over time, or with treatment, the clinically distinct features of the primary cicatricial alopecias become less distinct.
> In the end stage, characteristic features of these diseases are no longer present.

They become indistinguishable and look alike: bare patches coalesce into large bare areas devoid of follicular ostia and devoid of inflammation.

> One exception: DLE in the late or end stage can be distinguished by the hypo- and hyperpigmentation of the scalp and ears and follicular plugging in the ears.
> A note of caution: Be careful not to misdiagnose a patient with acute stage PPB or CCCA as having end stage-disease because of the absence of symptoms or signs.
> In PPB and CCCA, clinical spreading and extent of inflammatory infiltrate (in a scalp biopsy) may be the only two indicators of ongoing activity and signal the need for treatment.

Suggested Reading

Headington JT. Cicatricial alopecia. Dermatol Clin. 1996;14:773–82.

Mirmirani P, Willey A, Headington JT, et al. Primary cicatricial alopecia: histopatholologic findings do not distinguish clinical variants. J Am Acad Dermatol. 2005;52:637–43.

Whiting DA. Cicatricial alopecia: clinico-pathological findings and treatment. Clin Dermatol. 2001;19:211–25.

Understanding and Helping Patients with Cicatricial Alopecia

As a physician, you can have a direct and profound impact on the lives of cicatricial alopecia patients who truly need your help. Even though we do not know yet the cause or have fully effective treatments or a cure for cicatricial alopecia, we urgently need doctors who are willing to better understand and treat patients and to provide compassionate and encouraging care.

The world's only voice for patients and families with cicatricial alopecia comes from the advocacy and support of the Cicatricial Alopecia Research Foundation (CARF), which is entirely devoted to finding the best treatments and the cure for these diseases. Until CARF was formed in 2004, patients with these rare conditions had nowhere to turn for information, support, and referrals to dermatologists with expertise in these disorders. CARF fills this need and provides the tools to heal the emotional effects of permanent hair loss.

On the following pages, you will read about the candid and touching journeys of patients who experienced difficulties in getting adequate diagnosis and treatment or who have been rejected and left feeling depressed and hopeless. With your assistance, this can change. In addition to being knowledgeable about the best treatment options available, physicians can play a significant role in helping patients cope with their disease by validating their concerns and by encouraging them to lead normal and fulfilling lives.

CARF invites you to become a partner and participate with our dedicated and successful team. We encourage you to sign up at our website, http://www.carfintl.org, for ongoing updates about cicatricial alopecia research.

We are grateful to Carol Kotroczo for her valuable administrative assistance. We also wish to thank Nancy FitzGerald for her sage advice and for editing this chapter.

On Fire for Research and a Cure!

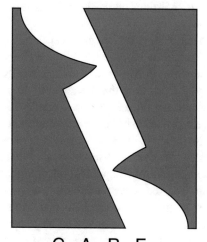

C . A . R . F .

The logo of CARF

V. Price and P. Mirmirani (eds.), *Cicatricial Alopecia: An Approach to Diagnosis and Management*, DOI 10.1007/978-1-4419-8399-2_10, © Springer Science+Business Media, LLC 2011

Cicatricial Alopecia Needs You!

Diagnosis: Lichen planopilaris

S.B

Drawing from my own experiences in grappling with cicatricial alopecia and from the retelling of fellow patients' journeys, it is obvious that many patients with cicatricial alopecia patients do not get a clear diagnosis, proper treatment, emotional support or current information about their disease.

My personal journey with cicatricial alopecia began more than 10 years ago. After seeing several dermatologists who could not give me a clear diagnosis, I arrived at the office of Dr. Vera Price without an appointment, desperate and in great pain, feeling as if pick axes were imbedded deep into my scalp. Dr. Price confirmed my diagnosis of LPP. She gave me the worst-case scenario: I would lose more hair and it would not grow back. I wept while Dr. Price comforted me. She said, "You'll get a partial hairpiece and no one will ever know." Little did I know then that our doctor-patient relationship would blossom into a friendship that would benefit cicatricial alopecia patients around the world.

After I attended an alopecia areata patient conference in Norfolk, Virginia and met 750 youngsters, many of whom had totally bald heads, I knew then that I wanted to help others who had my disease. Several months later, Dr. Price happened to be in Los Angeles and accepted my invitation to attend a brunch at my home for friends who wanted to learn about my hair loss. The strong show of support at this informal gathering was the springboard for our grassroots effort to promote research to find better treatments and a cure for cicatricial alopecia, and to support education and raise public awareness. Spurred by this, Dr. Price and I founded the CARF, which became a nonprofit organization in 2004. In its few short years, CARF has made extraordinary progress in funding ground breaking research and in educating both patients and the medical profession.

In spite of the strides we have made, patients still have a vital need for greater support, and this is where dermatologists can play a unique role. For most patients, it is emotionally devastating to learn that they have a disease that is painful, often accompanied with severe burning and itching, and causes permanent hair loss. Hair is an important part of our self-image! It takes time to adjust to this new and difficult situation.

Dermatologists are the only specialists with expertise to diagnose and treat hair loss in general and the cicatricial alopecias in particular. No other physicians are trained to recognize and manage this difficult group of permanent hair loss conditions.

Doctors and their staff can play a meaningful part in patients' education, acceptance, and recovery. Doctors and their staff can tell cicatricial alopecia patients about CARF, give them CARF brochures, and refer them to CARF's website at http://www.carfintl.org, where they can get up-to-date information.

We invite dermatologists and their staff to join our dedicated, successful team and become partners in helping patients receive better quality care. The commitment and support of the medical community would be an invaluable gift that would lift patients' spirits and help them feel whole again. Cicatricial alopecia needs you!

Looking in the Mirror

Diagnosis: Central Centrifugal Cicatricial Alopecia

G.P.T

"This is serious. Your scalp is like a sponge. It won't hold hair." These are the only words I remember hearing from the first dermatologist I went to see regarding my hair loss. These were the words he also used to describe a patient who was bald – a woman I happened to know. I don't remember much else. I was frozen all over. I maintained my composure until I reached the car, tearful and shaking, where all the emotion unloaded. I could barely breathe – "Serious… sponge!"

I went to the dermatologist after noticing a bare area on the crown of my head when combing my thick hair. Like many African-American women, I went to the hair salon bi-weekly. I had first asked my hair stylist about this thinning area during one of my visits and she told me it was just natural thinning from age. Finally, I developed the courage to "look in the mirror" and was *devastated*. I found a sizeable diamond-shaped area without hair. After seeing the dermatologist, there were periods of time when I could not think or feel. I just kept looking in the mirror to make sure my "sponge" was covered with my longer hair.

I went to see a second dermatologist who, in contrast to the first doctor, gave me a little more hope. She had me look in the mirror again and showed me that some hair follicles were still there, while they were not present in other places. She said I needed a biopsy and referred me to an international specialist, Dr. Vera Price.

Dr. Price examined me, explained what was needed for a proper diagnosis and performed a painless biopsy. She explained the nature of the biopsy and why she chose what looked like the most recently affected area. While I did not tell her about "the sponge" and did not understand everything she said, she gave me confidence that she was indeed an expert and knew what she was doing. She explained the different types of alopecia, what they looked like, and the different growth patterns. When I returned for my follow-up visit, she confirmed the diagnosis of cicatricial alopecia (scarring alopecia). Although I was sorely disappointed, I felt assured that her diagnosis was accurate.

During the same visit, she asked a question that was far from my mind: "How are you going to maintain a beautiful hair style?" Beauty and scarring alopecia – what an oxymoron! However, along with starting a treatment regime of Plaquenil, Kenalog injections, and scalp topicals, I began pondering her question. She explained that the main focus of my hair care was to be as gentle as possible, and minimize the use of harsh chemicals on my hair to minimize hair breakage. I went back to my second doctor (an African-American female) who then referred me to another hair stylist.

The new hair stylist played a very important role in my adjustment to this disorder as she helped me to think about what I needed to do in order to maintain my appearance. I shared Dr. Price's comments with her. The stylist and I decided to eliminate the use of chemicals to straighten my hair and to use *only* semipermanent color. She created a natural style that suited my face. Visit after visit, she reinforced the beauty of my tight natural curls.

As a facilitator/teacher, I teach others to "look in the mirror" to see the deepest "why" of their behavior and to see who they really are – not who they have become. Each day I also look in the mirror to see if the areas without hair are properly covered. One day I realized that I was always looking in the mirror at my hair, but what I really needed to do was to look in the mirror at *me. Who am I? What is my deepest why? What defines me?* Over a period of time, my self-examination revealed:

* It is normal to grieve a loss…including hair loss
* I am not my hair. I am an African-American woman with faith, intellect, a friendly disposition, kindness, an analytical mind, and a consensus-building nature
* I developed an appreciation of my *natural* hair
* It could always be worse…just look around at other people
* What happens to me is part of *my life-journey*
* What people see is a brief chapter of that journey
* I am concerned about this disease of "NO" – there is no cure, no definitive treatment and no clear link to other diseases (which could provide a root cause)
* The CARF has been *the* vital avenue for maintaining updated information, providing support, helping others, and advocacy

My journey continues as my cicatricial alopecia has spread and I have occasional burning and itching. I have been on several different treatment regimes and continue to adjust to my reality. One of the biggest challenges has been my move across the country and finding a doctor who treats patients with hair loss. This time I knew what to look for in a physician and a hair stylist – someone who was knowledgeable about hair and cicatricial alopecia but also willing to continue to learn as the treatment process changes. Perhaps what matters most is the attitude my physician displays – that "we are on top of this as much as we can be with the limited current knowledge about cicatricial alopecia."

When I talk with others, I share my journey and encourage them to find a knowledgeable, caring physician and to learn how to care for themselves – both their hair/scalp as well as their emotional well-being. It is important for them to know that they, too, can move from devastation to hope and from despair to "looking in the mirror." What a journey!

My Hair Loss Encounter

Diagnosis: Frontal Fibrosing Cicatricial Alopecia

I.J

The first time I became aware that I had a hair loss problem was almost 8 years ago following the birth of my youngest child. My eyebrows suddenly became very sparse and were beginning to disappear.

As I had just given birth, I initially disregarded the problem, assuming that the stress upon the body caused by pregnancy and childbirth had caused me to lose some hair. I expected the problem to resolve over time. My father's battle with cancer and his subsequent death added to the stress. Months after the continued eyebrow sparseness, I noticed that my hair was becoming increasingly thin and difficult to manage. It had become very fine and fly-away and I was having difficulty making it look presentable. Still I accepted this as a temporary problem, assuming that we all go through these phases with our hair at various times in our lives.

After 2 years of progressive thinning of the hair, I moved with my husband and children from our home in England to America to begin a new job. It was at this time that I became more aware that the problem was getting worse. On my infrequent visits back home, my family would see a noticeable change that my hair was disappearing rapidly. At my mother's insistence, I decided to seek medical attention and was referred to my first dermatologist.

The dermatologist told me I was suffering from alopecia areata and mentioned female-pattern baldness. He advised me that the only treatment available was to inject steroids into my eyebrows, which he began. He instructed me to return for more of the same if the treatment proved effective. He also told me to start applying topical minoxidil to the scalp, morning and night, for the foreseeable future. I began to do this immediately and continued religiously for about 6 months. I did not return for further injections into the eyebrows as I could see no discernable improvement.

After 6 months of applying minoxidil, I decided to stop, as I could see no hair regrowth. By this time, my hair was not only thinning, but was receding back from the hairline at the forehead and extending to the temples. I gradually accepted the condition of my hair. I had tried the only treatment recommended to me without success and thought that now I would have to make the best of this condition.

I was referred to an endocrinologist. After a series of blood tests, he concluded that my hair loss was not due to an endocrine disorder and referred me to a second dermatologist. The new doctor was a young woman who confirmed a diagnosis of frontal fibrosing cicatricial alopecia after biopsies were taken from the scalp. I began steroid injections into the affected areas and was also referred to a dermatologist specializing in hair loss. After 11 months of steroid injections and taking the drug Plaquenil in an attempt to halt the hair loss process, the doctor and I agreed that this treatment did not appear to have been effective and so the injections were stopped.

My hair had become so thin and sparse (all the way back to the middle of the crown) that it was almost impossible to style it in a way that would cover the bare areas of my scalp. Running concurrently with my hair loss was the gradual erosion of my self confidence which had reached an all time low. To other people, describing myself as being "devastated" by the problem probably seems overly dramatic. I feel guilty for feeling sorry for myself due to my misfortune when there are people all over the world with serious illnesses. However, I can honestly say that losing my hair has had a detrimental effect on every aspect of my life. It occupies my thoughts in a negative way every single day.

On a more positive note, I recently returned from a clinic in London which specializes in hair systems specifically for people with varying degrees of hair loss. I had some hair extensions strategically placed to give the appearance of a fuller head of hair. I am so pleased with the results and I no longer have the feeling that people are looking at my scalp. It feels like a weight has been lifted from my shoulders. Despite the cost and need for regular maintenance of the hair system, I am pleased to have found a cosmetic solution to a problem that had badly dented my self-confidence. I plan to use it until current medical research can find a suitable treatment or cure for my condition.

Looking for Answers

Diagnosis: Folliculitis Decalvans

J.A

Ten years ago at age 45, I thought I would have a full head of hair indefinitely. With a background in the pharmaceutical industry, I felt I had beaten my family history of androgenetic alopecia. I had been using both minoxidil and finasteride for years before they were commercially available for hair growth and my hair looked great.

One morning in 1999, however, I noticed that my scalp was red and becoming more irritated by the day. When I saw angry-looking pustules, I quickly made an appointment with my dermatologist. Various shampoos and topical lotions did nothing, so I did some research. I learned about scarring alopecias, recognized the classical symptoms of folliculitis decalvans, and found a medication regimen that was shown effective in a British study. (That regimen remains the standard for folliculitis decalvans today and is described elsewhere in this monograph).

After visiting more than six different dermatologists, none would prescribe the medications I needed. At that time, very few knew how to diagnose cicatricial alopecia and even fewer understood the aggressive treatments required. I was very frustrated. I knew how I could be treated and could only go from physician to physician and find none who understood the disorder sufficiently to help me.

Many men with hair loss have the option of just being bald and shaved heads are even considered fashionable today. Certainly with androgenetic alopecia being so common, you might think that only the most vain man would be so concerned about hair loss. But my condition was different. Folliculitis decalvans – unlike more common alopecias and even some cicatricial alopecias where the scarring is below the surface of the skin – left my scalp visibly scarred.

I finally found a dermatologist willing to treat me and I have managed to keep at least a little of my hair through the many relapses and remissions over the last 10 years. I discovered Dr. Vera Price and the CARF. I only wish CARF had existed 10 years ago. Not only is CARF promoting awareness about cicatricial alopecia – and importantly, how to treat it – but I have met many other patients through CARF who have given me a great deal of support and perspective about my own situation.

Unfortunately, many of the fellow patients I meet still experience years of delay before their condition is correctly diagnosed and even longer before it is treated with effective medications. Time is critical in treating cicatricial alopecias. These conditions cause irreversible damage and they must be treated early and aggressively to prevent further hair loss and scarring. If treated early, many patients are able to keep enough hair to camouflage their condition. Sadly, many are only able to find effective treatments when it is too late to prevent a permanent impact on their appearance.

Any disorder that makes a person uncomfortable about the way he or she looks, in addition to being uncomfortable in the literal sense, can have a profound effect on one's self esteem. I have met people whose cicatricial alopecia has prevented them from realizing their potential in relationships, careers, and other vital aspects of their lives. With the information we have today, the frustrating experiences I had a decade ago should no longer be the norm. However, the people I continue to meet are still being diagnosed and treated too late. The readers of this monograph can help cicatricial alopecia patients avoid lifelong physical and psychological harm. I recognize that most dermatologists will see only a handful of cases such as mine, but with proper education, they can learn to recognize the symptoms and signs and become more comfortable with the aggressive treatments that cicatricial alopecia requires.

Discovering that there is help, and doing my small part to advance CARF's mission, have been very encouraging and rewarding for me. I am hoping that one day I will no longer meet people whose damage to their scalp has also damaged their lives. The readers of this monograph can do more than provide medical treatment. They can change lives. There will always be medical conditions for which tears and anguish are appropriate, but cicatricial alopecia should not be one of them. The information in this monograph gives the field of dermatology the power to help me realize my dream of seeing fewer tears.

My CICAL Journal

Diagnosis: Lichen Planopilaris

M.C

It began with red scaly areas on both sides of my scalp. Since there was no itching or discomfort, I was not overly concerned. I did not initially realize (although it became apparent over the next six months) that the disease process was already active in multiple sites and I had an enlarging area on the top of my head that was becoming progressively bald. So I began my journey into the world of cicatricial alopecia, which can best

be described as a roller coaster of clinical events and emotions.

I was initially diagnosed with alopecia areata. However, certain features of my presentation did not quite fit and I was referred to a "hair expert," Dr. Andrea Willey, who was the chief resident in the Dermatology Department at the University of Minnesota. She had gained expertise in the area during her hair research fellowship with Dr. Vera Price at the University of California, San Francisco, CA. If I had to identify the one person (or event) that made the difference in my journey, it would be this woman. To her credit, Dr. Willey determined that my proper diagnosis *was lichen planopilaris* and facilitated the transfer of my care and treatment plan to Dr. Maria Hordinsky, an esteemed dermatologist at the University of Minnesota with extensive experience treating cicatricial alopecia. She introduced me to the CARF and Sheila Belkin, CARF CEO, who guided and supported me through the painful period of accepting and coping with the realities of this disease which is, as Sheila states, "life-altering but not life-threatening."

Hair loss is disfiguring and our cultural mores about baldness range between acceptance (in certain situations) to the expectation that hair pieces or wigs are available to be used as needed. My hair was thin and high-maintenance, but it was a primal part of my identity. Watching the bald spots expand over the course of the next 2 years was devastating. Only a few people knew the true extent of my despair. As a scientist, I understood the inflammatory and immune aspects associated with cicatricial alopecia, but it did not mean I could accept my diagnosis. Therefore, I embarked on both a functional wellness program and a dedicated treatment plan to try to arrest the inflammatory process and save whatever hair I could.

What happened next was "the event" that totally changed the way I learned to cope with my disease. Due to a unique set of circumstances, I became immersed in the planning and production of a CARF Patient and Doctor Conference in Minneapolis. It allowed me to meet other patients with cicatricial alopecia, become better informed about the work being done to understand the pathophysiology of these diseases, and acquire the perspective and strength to discuss and handle my condition with a sense of self-confidence and optimism.

As I look back on my journey with cicatricial alopecia, I no longer ask "why me?" I am immensely grateful for the care and support that I have received. I attribute my progress to my *Three C Care Plan*: (1) correct diagnosis, (2) commitment to the treatment plan, and (3) CARF. As a scientist, I know that research is the key to the cure. As a patient, I know what it feels like to be diagnosed with an orphan disease. Therefore, I am indebted to the patients (including their families and friends) and the physicians and corporate groups who have extended themselves for those of us in need while the challenges of these diseases are pursued. Because of these efforts and dedicated funding, I am not alone on this journey.

A Call to Action: When in Doubt, Biopsy

Diagnosis: Central Centrifugal Cicatricial Alopecia

M. P-l

As a young woman with central centrifugal cicatricial alopecia (CCCA), more than just my hair has changed over the last few years. What started out as a small bare area on my right crown that was the size of a half dollar (easily hidden by my neck-length relaxed hair) has morphed into multiple bare areas covered by fuller adjacent kinky strands on a head of short natural hair. The experiences prior to and following my diagnosis transformed my life personally, socially, and professionally. Collectively, these experiences fueled a passion inside of me to learn more about hair disorders and to increase awareness of these conditions.

Before my condition took its rampant and increasingly painful course, I had been a medical student proud of the profession I had chosen but unsure of how I would best serve my community as a physician. Now I am a senior medical student who seeks to enter the field of dermatology with a desire to contribute to hair research and management of hair disorders. The ambiguity and frustration I experienced on my own path to diagnosis has led me to want nothing more than to educate patients and physicians alike about these poorly understood conditions that can be so devastating to patients and their loved ones. The paucity of research and adequate treatment options, coupled with the permanence of the condition, present a challenge to even the most experienced dermatologist.

It took several dermatology visits over a 2-year period to arrive at my diagnosis of CCCA. In retrospect, I had gone to well-qualified dermatologists who were hindered mostly by their lack of familiarity with my chronic hair condition, which appeared unlike any particular infectious process or nonscarring alopecia. Furthermore, I was physically healthy and had no known underlying conditions associated with hair loss. Thus, there was a hesitancy to perform a scalp biopsy. Since physicians aim to do no harm under the Hippocratic Oath, I understand the decision to avoid an invasive test and to simply treat empirically. However, due to its progressive nature and the permanence of the hair loss in cicatricial alopecia, it may be best to aggressively seek a diagnosis when the clinical picture or a lengthy hair loss history suggests a primary hair disorder, even if unfamiliar to the clinician. For me, my diagnosis came abruptly. With the hair loss areas enlarging and my scalp pain no longer amenable to topical steroids, an astute resident physician suggested I have a scalp biopsy.

Following my diagnosis, I read fervently as much as I could about cicatricial alopecia. My newfound awareness led me to encourage my mother to have a scalp biopsy. She had been suffering from progressive and painful hair loss for nearly 8 years. After much discomfort, embarrassment and depression from having lost most of her hair, my mother gained peace of mind from a biopsy that also confirmed CCCA. While it was too late to prevent further hair loss, it was an enlightening victory for both of to us to learn that we both had CCCA. The diagnosis brought awareness, closure, and an acceptance that we had both been missing before the biopsies were taken. My elation was heightened by my discovery of CARF, an organization wholeheartedly devoted to raising awareness, funding research, and advocating for those with cicatricial alopecia.

As a permanent hair loss disorder, cicatricial alopecia currently has no cure or definitive treatments to effectively control the hair loss. Cicatricial alopecia can involve a painful course, with individuals experiencing scalp pain, burning, itching, or tingling/crawling sensations that can ultimately impact physical and psychological health. Even if not symptomatic, the destructive hair loss alone is usually distressful enough to patients. A higher index of suspicion for cicatricial alopecia and early recommendation for a scalp biopsy to confirm the

diagnosis may help alleviate much of the uncertainty that surrounds these inflammatory and irreversible conditions.

Takeaway Pearls

> Patient experiences highlight the impact that the cicatricial alopecias have on the lives of patients
> The distress and devastation caused by the hair loss is heard over and over and stresses the importance of the physician's validation and compassion
> A scalp biopsy is the first step in diagnosis and management: if you suspect a cicatricial alopecia, take a biopsy
> Cicatricial alopecias are not hereditary. The one exception is CCCA that may occur in other family members, usually women

Index

V. Price and P. Mirmirani (eds.), *Cicatricial Alopecia: An Approach to Diagnosis and Management*,
DOI 10.1007/978-1-4419-8399-2, © Springer Science+Business Media, LLC 2011

Printed in the United States
By Bookmasters